Calm
Healing

141769

Calm Healing

Methods for a
New Era of Medicine

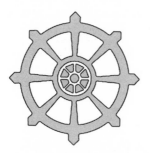

Robert Bruce Newman

Ruth L. Miller

North Atlantic Books
Berkeley, California

Published by
North Atlantic Books
P.O. Box 12327
Berkeley, California 94712

Cover and book design by Paula Morrison
Printed in the United States of America

Calm Healing is a registered trademerk of Medigrace, Inc., and the book title is used with the permission of Medigrace.

Excerpts from *Transpersonal Medicine* by G. Frank Lawlis, copyright © 1996 by G. Frank Lawlis. Reprinted by arrangement with Shambhala Publications, Inc.

Calm Healing: Methods for a New Era of Medicine is sponsored by the Society for the Study of Native Arts and Sciences, a nonprofit educational corporation whose goals are to develop an educational and crosscultural perspective linking various scientific, social, and artistic fields; to nurture a holistic view of arts, sciences, humanities, and healing; and to publish and distribute literature on the relationship of mind, body, and nature.

Library of Congress Cataloging-in-Publication Data

Newman, Robert Bruce, 1935–
    Calm healing : methods for a new era of medicine / Robert Bruce Newman and Ruth L. Miller ; foreword by Richard Grossinger.
        p. ; cm.
    Includes bibliographical references and index.
    ISBN-13: 978-1-55643-626-0 (pbk.)
    ISBN-10: 1-55643-626-2 (pbk.)
    1. Mind and body therapies. 2. Alternative medicine. I. Miller, Ruth L., 1948– II. Title.
    [DNLM: 1. Mind-Body and Relaxation Techniques. 2. Mental Healing. WB 880 N554c 2006]
RC489.M53N49 2006
616.89'1—dc22

2006026675

1 2 3 4 5 6 7 8 9 VERSA 12 11 10 09 08 07 06

The species sees itself alive and growing fast
With so much deadly might in its power
It turns faster into the light of its mass

REFERRING TO THE BODY OF HUMANITY and the light that makes up all human bodies, multidimensional bodies of light, the words above describe the essence of the methods we are presenting in this book. From the point of view of the quantum sciences, all bodies are composed of dynamic units of space in which electrons blaze. Their charged substance comes into and burns out of time and space at extremely high speed, leaving overlapping brilliant traces. But even more fundamental to our living bodies is a light that is far more brilliant and powerful than the radiant activity of the atoms. Some physicists see that we are founded in "boundless luminosity,"[1] an inherent characteristic of space itself. This fundamental light has various dimensions active in the plenum of space and has been spoken of as dimensions of inner light inherent in the human body. In the revered literature of the spiritual sciences the ultimate inner light, the supreme potential of human function, is called "undiminishing luminous clarity"[2] or "the ground luminosity."[3] And in the moment before death, when the tendencies of the lifetime have dissolved, this supremely life-giving light

1. Mark Cummings, *The Courage to Change* (Nevada City, CA: Joy, 2004), 31.
2. Dudjom Rinpoche, *Dudjom Tesar Ngondro* (New York: Yeshe Melong, 1984), 31.
3. Sogyal Rinpoche, *The Tibetan Book of Living and Dying* (San Francisco: HarperSanFrancisco, 1994), 256.

is revealed as the light of life itself.[4] Our moment in history, the early twenty-first century, is characterized by an increasing unity of spiritual science and physical science and an accelerating realization of the true nature of the body. This new model of the human body, appropriate for today's new methods of therapy and diagnosis, is a body that is, truly, turning faster into the light of its mass.

4. Ibid., 255; also referred to by various Christian mystics and shamans.

Contents

Foreword by Richard Grossinger ix

Introduction xxiii

Part One: Meditation and Mind-Body Medicine

Chapter 1. Mind-Body Medicine Comes of Age. 3

Chapter 2. Meditation Methods Across Cultures. 25

Chapter 3. Meditation Research in the United States 45

Part Two: A New Model for Healing

Chapter 4. States of Consciousness—Emerging
Understandings. 83

Chapter 5. A New Model of the Body for a New Era of
Medicine 103

Chapter 6. A New Model of the Healing Process 143

Part Three: Healing Methods

Chapter 7. Cardio-Awareness Healing Systems. 165

Chapter 8. Progressive Neuromuscular Release 173

Chapter 9. Awareness-Based Energy Breathing. 193

Chapter 10. Transformative Compassionate Breathing. 207

Chapter 11. Applications Around Childbirth 219

Chapter 12. Healing the Present by Healing the Past. 253

Chapter 13. The Healing Practice of Humor 277

Chapter 14. Health Care Methods for the Semi-Comatose
and Comatose, and for Near-Death Care. 289

Part Four: New Possibilities

Chapter 15. Transforming Our Paradigm of Illness 311

Chapter 16. Healing the Person, Healing the Planet 317

Chapter 17. The Genius of Self-Care 329

Appendix: The Light Nature of the Energy Body
According to *Vajrayana* Buddhism 335

Concise Bibliography of *Vajrayana* Literature in English 340

Glossary 342

Index 350

Acknowledgments 361

About the Authors 364

Foreword

By Richard Grossinger

THIS BOOK IS A CLEAR MAP to the evolution of a new paradigm, not only of healing but of living.

Esoteric astronomer Rodney Collin wrote the following in his journal in 1955: "When a new gift, a new possibility, is given to the earth, it is always presented in two ways, in unconscious form, and in conscious form. In the hydrogen bomb we recognize the unconscious form of a power hitherto unknown on earth. We await the demonstration of the same power in conscious form, that is, incarnate in living beings."*

Around the same time, French anthropologist-priest Pierre Teilhard de Chardin spoke of an inertial power equivalent to gravity, more transmogrifying than any weapon or machine: "Someday, after mastering the winds, the waves, the tides, and gravity, we will harness for God the energies of love. And then, for the second time in the history of the world, humankind will have discovered fire."

Switch the topic from physics to medicine, and the same ratio lies within lasers, ultrasound and magnetic resonance machines, and molecularized drugs: we await their conscious form, and it will be something akin to conscious transference, by the medium of self-less love.

---

*Rodney Collin, *The Theory of Conscious Harmony* (London: Robinson & Watkins Books, Ltd, 1958), p. 191.

In whatever direction our species goes, if humanity is to benefit from the centuries of scientific knowledge and technological development without, at the same time, becoming trapped in its gulag of cybernetic machines or subjugated by its oracle of genetic determinism and sold out to its pharmaceutical monopolies, people must begin to understand that their bodies are their own, their health is their own, and they are their own best physicians.

Right now we are clueless. We straggle through labyrinths of biological bodyshops and automotive clinics for people who are cell-based robots, hospitals that are assembly lines and garbage transfer stations.

Once people are mere commodities, to themselves and their physicians, they lose their vivacity. Having generated capital, they are expendable. But human beings are cosmic power stations, incipient Jedi knights; lamas and magicians—living alchemy. Neither the medical nor the pharmaceutical industries, trapped in myopic world-views and socioeconomic agendas that are too vast for even their denizens to perceive, have a clue of this. Like hooded birds, they see only what they are supposed to see. And they assume that they are right; their way, the only way.

We need to reclaim the shamanic, vitalistic, psychosomatic, yogic basis of healing and self-healing because we are suffering an epidemic of iatrogenic and agrogenic disease (pathologies caused by, respectively, physicians and food), and because materialist medicine is taking away not only people's basic health but their hope, their intrinsic healing capacity, their compassion for their own bodies (and those of others), and their destinies as angelic entities and alchemical beings.

As long as we profess and practice ignorance about our own body-minds and do not find or develop their intrinsic healing capacities, we forfeit the wonder and miraculous self-organizing, transformative core of our existence in this incredible universe. We squander it through our trance of clever, hegemonous imaging devices; reductionist-fundamentalist preachers in the guise of doctors, defending dogmas of academic medicine and its trade association; HMO managers and insurance-company executives for whom the patient is a gull in a profit-and-loss equation; and drug pushers combining the worst of Aldous Huxley's *Brave New World* (pills yielding lifetimes of artificial bliss) with the worst of George Orwell's *1984* (an authoritarian state run by royal elites and military-industrial lobbies and their captive politicians).

The simplest choice now, the only choice, is for people to begin to learn how to take responsibility for their own well-being—in short, their own lives—to reclaim their innate capacities for transduction and transubstantiation, for cellular internalization and telekinesis.

This crossroads is a subset of a greater global crisis, otherwise known as: "utopia or apocalypse," transformation or oblivion. The only alternative to becoming no one and nothing, a slave of staggeringly powerful, arrogant cabals, is to become someone and something, a magician able to heal not only himself or herself but others, someone able to change the direction of civilization.

There is a paradox. The material model of medicine is in ascendance. It is dominating the United States and, through cultural and economic globalization, the world. Yes, material medicine has made astonishing breakthroughs into understanding the biophysical, biochemical, and genetic processes shaping life: our metabolism, development, and the etiology of some (but not all) disease predispositions and trajectories. Along with this knowledge has come a vector-specific delivery system for cures (almost always either pharmaceutical or surgical). The American Medical Association and its affiliates among transnational pharmaceutical and petrochemical guilds export this concrete medicine and its accoutrements to the rest of the planet. It comes in a well-known package, along with Hollywood movies, Monsanto's chromosomes, the American dollar, and neocon propaganda about democracy. It would appear that it is the only health game in town.

At the same time, this great medicine machine is failing. It is failing economically because health is not a commodity and cannot be parsed and calculated into profits.

It is failing ethically because it is tied to a horrid HMO/insurance system that has as its primary goal (nonetheless) generating corporate profits at the price of real medicine.

But, *most significantly*, it is failing at an ontological level because it is tied to a scientism which premises that existence is mechanical and molecular in a static, linear way. Even its famously dynamic physiology and microbiology are static and linear, for they leave consciousness and existential being out of their formulae.

No one would question the scope of the achievement of science in the context of its investigation into each and every cellular apparatus and network. But that achievement is itself framed by the goal that researchers and physicians have set: to reduce life and its healthy functioning to naked material parameters and then to address these in absolute technological terms. Under this regime a cell has to be a concrete entity rather than a fluid field through which matter and energy flow and are transmuted.

When the tools for diagnosis and treatment are robots, the person being treated is also a robot or, more precisely, only the part of an individual that is robot-like is being treated. Western medicine is based on keeping all supposedly metaphysical influences out. The devastating term "quackery" snatches in its octopus reach anything that intimates that 1). mind can influence matter in any way; 2). life has a synergistic element that includes consciousness; or 3.) states of being translate into states of health or disease.

Doctors additionally want their patients to be passive and *acted upon* and not to *act* upon their conditions, even in complementary procedures and practices alongside the dominant treatment mode. That is not to say that physicians are unaware of the role of lifestyle, diet, emotional states, etc., in health and disease, but even most of the hip ones have predetermined a material context for these things too and use them, relative to their actual potency, at a hierarchical level equivalent to—using science's own metaphor—stone tools vis-à-vis cyclotrons.

And yet, while the material paradigm is in the ascendance, a new paradigm is emerging and spreading like wildfire. It is both post-modern and ancient, eliciting elements of shamanic healing and psychic projection as old, probably, as the original massage, divination, and herbal sodalities of the Palaeolithic epoch—and with influences as multicultural and regionally diverse as early Buddhist meditation, *yoga*, *chi gung*, palpation, ceremonial visualization, sand-paintings, meditation in ice caves, therapeutic drumming and blowing, and uncountable other practices from every continent.

The new paradigm is post-modern in its reapplication of scientific analysis and empiricism to such activities as nonsectarian meditation, prayer, and faith healing; psychic projection and transference, placebo effects; conscious breathing; and psi phenomena (including telekinesis), all of which are elements of an emerging nonmaterial medicine.

It is post-modern in another sense: the provisional paradigms emerging from relativity theory, quantum mechanics, string theory, dark matter, and the like provide better models for understanding what is happening in body-minds than the traditional rubrics of Newtonian thermodynamics.

The new paradigm also encompasses a wide range of recently developed (or reconfigured) modalities such as *Reiki*, Bach Flower remedies, homeopathy (e.g. nanopharmacology), Polarity, biofeedback, and cranial osteopathy. What these systems and techniques share is a commitment to using our status as minded creatures to influence our states of health and cellular equilibrium and to catalyze our natural self-healing and homeostasis.

Nonmaterial medicine is not a rival to material medicine. It is truly its partner. Matter can't always be transmuted or transduced by mind, so drugs and scalpels are necessary too. But, in the long run, taking economics, ecology, and societal well-being into the equation, we will do much better to ignore technological medicine than we will to ignore the syncretic modality that Robert Newman and Ruth Miller aptly call "calm healing."

"Calm healing," not "Bones" McCoy's hand-held doctoring device in *Star Trek*, is the best hope for the future of medicine. After the decline of global petroleum civilization, the Earth will likely experience a version of "calm healing" through the reinvestiture of regional and local healers.

Material preemption or intervention is always an option, and its science, now that it has been birthed and refined, will probably be locked into the human enterprise in one form or another for its duration. "Calm healing," however, is even more fundamental; it is our birthright and, for the long haul—the haul past the age of petroleum and climate change—it has the greater potential for healing not only people but people in environments, environments themselves, and multiple species, e.g. whole ecosystems.

The "calm healing" model proposes, among other things, that mind is neither a mere epiphenomenon nor a languid prisoner of body; it is the necessary and absolute nucleus of vital embryogenesis through which a body assembles itself nonlinearly as holograms in fractal space. It conditions—in the sense of creating conditional reality—and molds bodies into their living, self-organizing, inherently mutating state. Big mind (as opposed to the monkey chatter of gossip mind) is always present as a potential active force in organismic state change. It is as much a fact of nature as water or *roches moutonnées*, those immense glacial boulders on the tundra of little mind.

The notion that mind over matter and intuitive faith are, by definition, futile "wishful thinking," is a ludicrous misjudgment and underestimation of the paraphysics of thought. An individual's health crisis is virtually always catalyzed—and often initiated as well—by wishing *too little*, by shutting off the force of mind, of invocation, of prayer, of mantra, of intention, or by damning them with faint-hearted use.

No, a mere wishy-washy wish is not going to cure or energetically imbue serious disease. It is the kind of dynamic wish that a shaman or faith-healer learns to conduct which has the accuracy and impact of a laser beam, the atomized force of a star. The science of this mode of projection lies in the turbulent zone between traditionary magic and chaos/complexity dynamics.

Through observation of the body of creation, through painstaking development of metonymical and microcosmic techniques, through inculcation in his/her being by (sometimes) fifty thousand or more repetitions,* a shaman concentrates, packages, and delivers a wish. He literally transfers it, in a manner Freud rediscovered as the therapeutic art of psychotherapy in a Western lineage. He accomplishes this transference probably instantaneously, if not (*mirabile dictu!*) at a speed even greater than light in a measurable sense—or, more accurately, in a mode that has nothing to do with either speed or chronology.

We need to wish more sincerely, more sustainedly, with more specificity and a more conscious trajectory. We need to subtilize and entrain our mindedness so that it can tune to the realm of mitochondrial and Golgi function—what radical osteopath John Upledger calls "cell talk" and matrilineal therapists Bonnie Bainbridge Cohen and Emilie Conrad teach in the form of internalized movements that, at least symbolically, intercept the highly discrete realm of tissues and organs, lysosomes and organelles.

When the Everly Brothers sang, *"Only trouble is, gee whiz, I'm*

---

*Not all "calm healing" modes are this active, of course, only those that gain their power from sincere repetition. The rationale of all those practices (involving repetition or not) is this: a magician/martial artist who knows what it feels like to be in the ring with a dangerous opponent will not get stage fright and tremble at the presence of spirits or equivocate at the moment of truth. She will have learned her movements so profoundly that she will just do them, no matter the opponent, no matter the fog of cynicism all about her.

dreaming my life away," they were serenading the troubadour of passive dreaming, of unrequitable longing. Robert Newman and Ruth Miller are heralding another kind of dreaming, active and lucid — active, lucid praying; active, lucid visualizing. This is accessible to a practitioner only after honing her receptivity and sensitivity and doing the necessary fifty thousand or so preparations. It is to dream one's life back and not away.

Conversely, even a million repetitions will accomplish nothing without concomitant internalization, which means gradually cultivated and deepened awareness.

There is also a quantum element, in the sense of both uncertainty principle and the quantum leap that can, in a moment of pure, intentional faith, skip the repetitions and go straight to the enlightened, illumined meaning of one/every thing. No doubt this is what is meant by the puissance of prayer. Quantum touch and tantric invocation permeate the teachings of Jesus of Nazareth, though most modern Bible-readers glide through the scriptures without getting it.

John Upledger discovered that, when therapists work with sick clients in the water accompanied by dolphins, these nonhuman "physicians" nuzzle the entry points to lesions and aim their sonar through blockages, malignancies, or (in Upledger's nomenclature) "energy cysts." The difference between an intuitive, living, biological sonar and a laboratory one is the difference between minded, directed elixir and unminded, robotic engineering. In the former, prayer and love are an active force. In the latter, no transference occurs, no synergistic ripple spreads, no deep internalizing cell-by-cell lotus unfolds; there is only budging the mule with a rope. The mule may move, but not much and not for long.

In 1972 Freudian-oriented parapsychologist Jule Eisenbud described to me the negative voodoo or hexing aspect of this same quantum mind-body physics: "Thoughts alone can kill; bare naked thoughts; isn't all this armor of war, this machinery, these bombs, aren't they all grotesque exaggerations? We don't even need them.

To put it schematically, and simplistically, and almost absurdly, because we don't wish to realize that we can just kill with our minds, we go through this whole enormous play of killing with such—, of overkilling with such overimplementation; it gets greater and greater and greater, as if … it's a caricature of saying: how can I do it with my mind? I need tanks; I need B-52 bombers; I need napalm, and so on, and so on."

Substitute "heal" for "kill" and make the equivalent substitutions throughout this polemic, and you have the first principle and axiom of a new model of medicine. In a flourish concluding his rant, Eisenbud echoes Freud: "All science has produced cover stories for the deaths we create; it's streptococci; it's accidents, and so on. But, what I'm trying to say is, there must be, I feel, a relationship between this truth, which we will not see, and this absurd burlesque of aggression that goes on all around us, as if we're trying to deny that the other is possible."

The response from the 'hood—in a not entirely unimaginable future, after crime clans and street gangs have turned into healing societies and shamanic lodges—hopefully is, "Right on, late brother!" Consider for a moment a civilization, a planet, that permitted and nurtured love bombers instead of death and suicide bombers; in which al-Qaeda, the base, trained guerrillas of therapeutic transformation who immolated disease-causing cysts of all kinds. I mean a planet from the bottom up, wherein sea squirts and worms exude medicine for other creatures, across which dolphins and bears teach healing rather than predation, in whose skies and fields hawks and mice exchange mantras and prayers.

It was never in the cards for us to transform nature or its primeval jungles, but instead it was possible long ago (and perhaps still is) to mutate nature totemically in men and women clad as warrior beasts empowered for curing as well as killing. It was always possible for lions and coyotes, for bad guys and witches to do good by bad. This is why the word "bad" now marks a conjunction of "good" and "bad," at which, alone, "good" has any real munition, any gumption. As the *chi gung* master/reggae priest is wont to chant, in these words or others, *"I'm gonna put on an Iron Shirt/and chase Satan off o'Earth."*

Of course, mullahs and terrorists aver that is the very deed they are enacting on the cancer of the crusader, blasphemous West: they are incinerating its tumor off the Earth. If Osama bin Laden taught an esoteric tarot, he might "communiqué" to the effect that, when his lightning in the form of hijacked jets struck the tower of ignorance, tyranny, and stale habit, it released seeds of conscious possibility. But whenever implacable machineries or explosives are employed in place of minded subtlety and compassion, only tragic things happen, only dread diseases result, and those diseases escalate into worse and more violent globalizing plagues.

This brings us to a second therapeutic principle of "calm healing": Whatever the healer, or the person acting wittingly or unwittingly as the healer, carries in his or her energy field—his propensity to his own illness, his vitality—is transmitted in some fashion to the patient insofar as patient and healer occupy and jointly activate the same "mutually containing field." I am drawing on the words and concepts of Edward Whitmont, a Jungian analyst who also practiced homeopathy. Universalizing the language of homeopathy, Whitmont postulated that the symbolic awareness of the healer (or destroyer) potentizes his or her "disease" (ideally, its healing potential) and transmits the medicine of his being, his divine wound. He either enhances the power of the organism to self-organize through the opportunity of the disease, to grow beyond its transient symptomology, or he further undermines the patient and deadens both organisms' innate synergistic potentiation, the doctor's as well as the patient's. A shaman or doctor (again, wittingly or unwittingly) stands in a role that allows him or her to become either a ratification of pathology (by overmaterialized beliefs and treatments) or a homeopathic simillimum, a vitalization of the disease through subtle energy and a reinstatement of the original morphogenic capacity of the life field.

The true healing function is epigenesis. The hex that stands against it is genetic determinism and despair—the belief that we are no more than elaborate, flawed machineries, barely able to repair but a few instrumentally prescribed vectors.

This second therapeutic principle leads to a third: the universe—all the star-ridden, quasar-ringed, black-hole way to its limitless limits in this dimension, beyond even the furthermost telescopically, radiationally magnifiable galaxies—is a field of life energies. These are available and assimilable.

While we clearly arise in a maelstrom of supernovas and runaway asteroids and comets, we also are receptors of a very high esoteric octave of energy. Beyond the random violence and debris of astrophysical space we are sacred, *prana*-filled, *chakra*-channel bodies. These two versions of the cosmos defy and contradict each other, but they also meld into the single cosmos in which we reside. In us physical and vital universes, macrocosm and microcosm ravel and converge. Sacred geography becomes sacred anatomy. Just because toxic radiations erupt and humongous, out-of-control objects predominate everywhere does not mean that healing energies, alchemical mutations, chi, and orgone do not also exist everywhere too, at a subtler and ultimately more profound level.

Picture a great moebius network of spirals opening out through a spout much like that of a ciliated microorganism, into the physical universe. A palpable externalized domain pours out of the fat end of the tube like a flood from a fire-hydrant spigot. At its tail, the spiral curls down into the finest, most gossamer thread, which winnows below the realm of atoms, quarks, and superstrings, drooling into dimensions of pure energy.

Outside our ordinary senses, beyond our dominant view of cosmic space, we are ever in another universe, another illumination, another thermodynamics, that, unlikely as this sounds, dwarfs the perceptible one by a factor of more than ten billion to one. In fact, matter is the flea that mind is scratching into existence.

It is from this transdimensional universe that efficacious energies of *Reiki*, faith-healing, simillima, therapeutic transduction, prayer, shamanic invocation, and millions of other practices across the diverse worlds of the universe are summoned—the great common vat.

The difference between the exoteric energy pool used by scientists (thus far) for their Star Wars and the subtle energy field tapped by healers and lamas is that the latter is not explicit or gross; it cannot be accessed by brute force or tyranny; it is cultivated, siphoned, and decanted only by subtle, disciplined techniques. Subtle energy is inaccessible, thank goodness, to the galaxies' soldiers and industrialists, as these would surely, if they could, harness it to the ends of subjugation of sentient beings, making the history of life the history of slavery. The real, enduring energy of creation is protected by a password, a code that can never be faked because it must be lived, is never merely provided, cannot be blackmailed or bluffed, yet is always available through the grace and sincerity of calm intentional, compassionate practices.

Newman and Miller have written a virtual bible of "calm healing," a primer for a new medicine. Not only have they explored its history and science, but they have created actual protocols and prayers—word-by-word incantations. Thus, this book is not only an account of a possibility. It is *the manual*, the starting point for practice. What we have here is a rare thing: phonemes that are things, statements that breathe medicines.

The reader should be warned, however, that "calm healing," despite its user-friendly appellation, is not something that is delivered effortlessly like a New Age balm. It is work. Pacifying and conducting consciousness takes focused yoga and committed attention/intention. It cannot happen idly or because we are nice people.

Its fruition, however, is the key to life on Earth, what ancient wisdom told us this planet is all about: working through consciousness to change the universe and do the work of God in the house of woman and man.

Richard Grossinger, publisher, North Atlantic Books; author of *Planet Medicine; Embryogenesis: Species, Gender, and Identity;* and *On The Integration of Nature: Post-9/11 Biopolitical Notes*

Introduction

THE WORLD CONSTANTLY CHANGES in its inconceivable dimensions and states, and in the twentieth century, change came more rapidly in more areas of life than ever before. In the midst of this speedy and extensive change, many aspects of human life have been transformed, and the field of medicine has experienced a paradigm shift.

Medical science as we know it, "scientific medicine," emerged in the late nineteenth century and flourished during World War II, when the advancement of surgical technology and pharmaceutical interventions led to an innocent confidence that modern scientific medicine could conquer all diseases and solve all health-related problems. This confidence was founded in experience: the remarkable results of high-technology surgery and the widespread demonstration of the effectiveness of antibiotics.

Scientific medicine is a powerful tool and a generally effective model, through which treatment of acute conditions such as injuries has most often been superb. But there has been a growing dissatisfaction with the prevalent use of drugs and surgery in response to a range of conditions, some of which may have benefited from another approach. Recently, the misuse and overuse of those interventions have become a significant problem, making hospital care one of the leading causes of death (American Medical Association 1998).

There is also growing concern about widespread addiction and reactions to various drugs, both prescribed and illegal. Anxiety and stress have become a pandemic psychophysical condition, engendering excessive dependence on drugs for "killing" pain and coping with unprecedented levels of psycho-emotional illness. As many as 90 percent of all office visits to doctors of conventional medicine during the 1980s and '90s were based on anxiety and stress (Benson 1996). Even the medical establishment is concerned about the high incidence of adverse drug reactions, with the American Medical Association reporting that reactions to prescriptions "may be the fourth to sixth leading cause of death" (American Medical Association 1998).

Through the twentieth century, scientific, or allopathic, medicine became characterized as a technological response to the body, and its practitioners were seen by patients and their families as too often lacking compassion. Doctors came to be seen as the victims of a limited and often restrictive medical training preoccupied with applying new drug protocols, largely defined by pharmaceutical corporations. Concern also emerged about the poor health of doctors and nurses, characterized by high rates of drug and alcohol addiction and shorter life spans than normal.

By the late 1990s, as a result of growing dissatisfaction with these potentially dangerous patterns, Americans were going to practitioners of Complementary and Alternative Medicine (CAM) more frequently than to providers of conventional medicine. Their distrust of established modes of health care and a desire for alternative modalities led to widespread interest in medical arts of other times and cultures, such as acupuncture, homeopathy, and herbal medicine, and in meditation science and mind-body therapies.

The reasons for the transfer of trust are multifold. CAM providers are typically healthier than establishment medical professionals and highly trained in the application of their specific modalities while understanding the limitations. They typically see themselves as healers and are very patient-oriented, intentionally sensitive to mind-body dynamics. Further, they spontaneously give both compassion and healing intention in the care they offer, which are pivotal values for the people seeking alternative health care.

In response to this movement, the U.S. National Institutes of Health has established a division of complementary and alternative medicine, and an increasing number of medical schools have begun to teach CAM modalities. These are signs that a significant shift is occurring in the medical paradigm. In his encyclopedic work, *Planet Medicine* (2000), Richard Grossinger offers a compelling vision of the scope and scale of the changes forthcoming. In the chapter called "The New Paradigm," Grossinger says:

> Paradigm shifts are elusive, multidimensional phenomena. In their midst no one can guess how far they will go and what they will eclipse ... Holistic health is finally a refraction of environmental awakening, political activism, and a synthesis of Eastern and Western epistemologies and ethics. It is not first and foremost a medical paradigm ... What passes now as "holistic health" or alternative medicine is merely the faintest glimmering of a new world. A new world will come anyway, as new worlds always have. This one, however, is millennial, not only because we are crossing the numerical millennium but because this is the historic moment at which progressive science and materialization of the planet have reached their physical limits. A new order must follow ... (538–41)

In her seminal description of the overall shift our culture is undergoing, *The Aquarian Conspiracy* (1980), Marilyn Ferguson offers a compelling description of the turning that is occurring in all aspects of American society—including the necessary revolution in the structure of medicine:

> If we respond to the message of pain or disease, the demand for adaptation, we can break through to a new level of wellness ... Just as the readiness of a new constituency makes a new politics, the needs of patients can change the practice of medicine ... a profession in which all people have a vital stake. (242–3)

The role of altered awareness in healing may be the single most important discovery in modern medical science. (250)

In 1993, Larry Dossey, MD, a brilliant internist, published his model of the "Three Eras of Medicine." In this model, Era I is scientific medicine, focused on observable "facts" and the diagnosis and elimination of symptoms, through suppression or surgery. Era II medicine, as defined by Dossey, is mind-body medicine, with its focus on methods that can help people take an active role in their health. Era III medicine, said Dossey, is transpersonal medicine, focused on methods that bring people to their innate abilities to heal themselves and others. As often happens during cultural shifts, all of these "Eras" are in place today. Era II and Era III medicine began to emerge simultaneously in America and the West in the 1970s and 1980s and continue to manifest and evolve today.

Another significant model of how the health sciences had to evolve is offered by Herbert Benson, whose decades of work at Harvard Medical School were pivotal to the emergence of some of the new medical methods. In his book, *Timeless Healing* (1996), Benson boldly stated that the scientific medical establishment would collapse under the weight of its own problems unless it developed a new model in which self-care was the essential feature. He proposed that if people were educated in the use of mind-body methods, such as meditation, they would be able to take an empowering role in their own health. Consequently, he suggested, pharmaceuticals and surgery would be used only as they supported self-care, which needs to be the primary mode of care.

In 1993, in *The Creation of Health*, Caroline Myss described the needed revolution in health care as a shift of power from the doctor to the patient. In the scientific medicine model of Era I, the doctor is all-powerful. In that model, the patient is passive and completely dependent on the doctor's directives, which, she says, is not a psychologically healthy situation for the patient (nor, we would submit, for the doctor!). To shift power from the doctor to the patient, health care education and training in mind-body methods would be key.

In parallel with these emerging new visions of possibility for the medical establishment, new understandings about the nature of the human body have emerged. Some of these realizations derive from the discoveries of other fields of science, such as quantum physics, cybernetics, electromagnetics, and biophysics. Others explain how it is that the CAM approaches are effective. Still other ideas emerge from our culture's discovery of the wisdom present in the time-tested practices of other cultures. Marilyn Ferguson was among the first to publish this knowledge in her 1980s journal, *Brain-Mind Bulletin*. Since then, many journals and organizations have continued to explore these alternatives, notably the Institute of Noetic Sciences, "New Dimensions Radio," Ken Wilber's numerous books, and the remarkable *Future of the Body* by Michael Murphy (1992).

It is presently 2006. This book presents a set of Era II and Era III methods developed over the past ten years—including methods that have been refined in application to cancer care, cardiovascular care, Alzheimer's care, near-death care, and childbirth. As of today, more than eighty training seminars in these methods have been presented in West Coast hospitals, all with education credits offered by the California Board of Registered Nursing. Several of the methods are applications of proven methods of meditation science. Other methods presented in this book are applications of the most proven methods of mind-body medicine, refined through many years of application. A few of the methods offer a new means of healing where, to date, no means that honor the emerging model of the human body have been available.

The chapters of this book present the background and context for these methods and verge into new theoretical domain. We explore the depths of the potential of self-care and the potential of human genius in healing. Our goal is to empower new dimensions of function by offering new ways to truly heal, to give birth, and to transform death into greater life. This work is a celebration, reclaiming great methods of inner wisdom from which our culture has been separated by materialist science, and presenting new methods to help the paradigm of medicine complete its shift into a more effective world of medical practice.

Most of the methods offered herein conform to Dossey's Era II model of medicine, but a few epitomize his Era III model. In hospital training programs offering the methods in this book, we have experienced a movement beyond individual health care to a new domain of group healing, in which emerging dimensions of healing potential have become evident through the powerful energies of intention. In these trainings people experience a practical knowledge of the unified field of which we all are a part, and express their intention to affect that field through personal healing and transformation—with often extraordinary results.

Intention has been known for millennia to have extraordinary power: individually and in groups, we are each the nucleus that brings forth the whole. So, with the effective action of groups engaged in mind-body healing, an exponential force for healing may be at hand. At the same time, our culture has achieved instantaneous worldwide communications via satellite, the computer, and telephone. The integration of these two factors brings us into a personal/global experience that holds the potential for worldwide mind-body healing.

The new medicine is immanent and long-awaited. It has the potential for mass healing—mass medicine—that can carry the individual practitioner into an unprecedented domain of well-being.

References

American Medical Association. News release. April 14, 1998.

Benson, Herbert. *Timeless Healing: Optimal Medicine, Optimal Health.* New York: Scribner, 1996.

Dossey, Larry. *Healing Words: The Power of Prayer and the Practice of Medicine.* New York: HarperCollins, 1993.

————. *Recovering the Soul*. New York: Bantam, 1989.

Ferguson, Marilyn. *The Aquarian Conspiracy*. Los Angeles: Tarcher, 1980.

Grossinger, Richard. *Planet Medicine*. Berkeley, CA: North Atlantic Books, 2000.

Murphy, Michael. *The Future of the Body: Explorations into the Further Evolution of Human Nature*. Los Angeles: Tarcher, 1992.

Myss, Caroline, and C. Norman Shealy. *The Creation of Health*. Walpole, NH: Stillpoint, 1993.

PART ONE

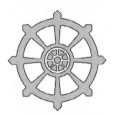

Meditation and Mind-Body Medicine

CHAPTER 1

Mind-Body Medicine
Comes of Age

FOR THOUSANDS OF YEARS, across human cultures, there has been an understanding that awareness—consciousness, soul, spirit, essence, whatever it may be called—is fundamental to all of existence, and that the human mind has an effect on both body and environment. The Platonic philosophers called it "idealism," stating that everything that seems to exist in the material world exists in potential outside of normal consciousness, to be called forth by the activity of mind. In the ancient *Vedic* traditions, the universe is described as energy, which, in Sanskrit, is called *Brahman,* condensed and organized into matter through consciousness. The several-thousand-year-old *Mundaka Upanishad* states:

> By energism of Consciousness Brahman is massed; from that Matter is born and from Matter, Life and Mind and the worlds.

This understanding is the basis for the Hindu and Buddhist principle that matter, with all the life-forms that have evolved within it, is *maya,* not truly real—because, ultimately, consciousness, or *Brahman,* is the only reality, and matter is a temporary form, maintained by the "energism," or energizing activity, of consciousness.

From Siberia to Mexico to Australia, shamans' journeys lead to the same conclusion: beyond the "worlds" of matter and illusion lies a reality beyond our perception, containing the potential of all possible forms of material existence. According to Carlos Castaneda, the Yaqui shaman Don Juan Matus, following ancient Toltec traditions, called that reality the *nagual*, and consistently warned Carlos to be careful, lest his own consciousness, unintended, create undesirable forms in the *nagual*.

Within these traditions, then, pure consciousness, or awareness—as distinct from thought—is a power: it manifests form out of the substance of the universe, in the body and outside it.

That Western science has not explored these ideas until recently is the result of a historical process in which study of the realm of spirit was assumed by the Church, with its theologians, and study of the physical world was given to "natural philosophers" and scientists. In medieval Europe, the Roman Catholic Church controlled dissemination of information and scholarship, which led to the persecution of Galileo and others for suggesting ideas that were not supported by the Church's cosmology. But the human search for knowledge is irrepressible. So, over several hundred years, through the Inquisition, the Renaissance, and into the period known as the Enlightenment, agreements were made and lines were drawn. Finally, they were clear: secular science could study matter and energy; the Church would still retain control over matters of spirit.

The split was formulated in the early 1600s, when René Descartes demonstrated to his and many others' satisfaction what became known as the "Cartesian split" between body and mind. He provided a rational justification for the Church to stick to its realm, leaving the increasing numbers of scientists the freedom to explore others. This tradition continued, and in fact was reinforced, through the Protestant Reformation, in which many new churches were formed on the premise that the Bible was the ultimate source of doctrine for all aspects of life. The "wall between church and state" set up by the U.S. Constitution's injunction that Congress would not "establish a religion" (that is, not set up a national, government-endorsed and supported church as was the norm in most of Europe) further reinforced the distinction between the two realms of inquiry.

It's only been since the power of the religious institutions has diminished, since the secularization of national and community life across Europe and the Americas, that science has dared to outwardly explore the realms of consciousness, or spirit. And it has only been in the twentieth century, when, unexpectedly, the new sciences of quantum physics and cybernetics made it essential to explore these areas, that the old injunction has finally fallen away. Not surprisingly, many people on both sides of the split—religion and science alike—are uncomfortable with this new realm of exploration, and some of them have spoken out against it as either "unscientific" or "of the devil."

Yet, today, the evidence is clear. In the very "hard" science of physics, it's been proved over and over again that all matter and energy is changeable: all possibilities exist at any moment, and the mind of the observer affects results. In the science of psychoneuroimmunology, a combination of anatomy, physiology, chemistry, psychology, and biophysics that emerged, in large part, out of research into the cause and cure of AIDS, the evidence demonstrates that the state of mind and emotions of the patient affect the activities of individual cells and the overall state of the body. In the science of cybernetics, the evidence shows that mind is just a part of the controlling mechanism for the body, functioning in many ways like a computer, but with measurable "emergent properties" that cannot be reproduced electronically, and that "self-organize" into the mind-body systems that make up all forms of life. Clearly, across the sciences, the union of body and mind can no longer be ignored.

The Unified Mind-Body

PERHAPS THE BEST-KNOWN ARTICULATOR of this union is Dr. Deepak Chopra, a Western-trained physician, former chief of staff of the New England Memorial Hospital, who came to understand, through the evidence presented to him in his practice, that there was far more to the healing process than his scientific background could explain. His first exploration of the potential for unification, entitled *Quantum Healing,* has become a classic. In it he traces his journey from a purely Western view of the body and mind as separate and unrelated, through quantum physics, and into the ancient traditions of the land of his birth. He describes his first inexplicable experience as occurring when he was an intern with an aged, dying man who had only days or hours to live, but who, when the youthful doctor Chopra blithely told him he'd see him when he returned from another assignment, held on to life for several weeks until his favorite doctor came and saw him again—and died almost immediately after. Chopra also tells the reverse kind of story, for example, the man who had lived comfortably with a tumor in his lungs for six years—until he was told it was cancer, at which point he became very upset and died shortly thereafter (1990).

Chopra explains these stories with the comment that our cells "are always willing to cooperate with the mind's instructions." He tells us, "The whole body is a 'thinking body,' the creation and expression of intelligence" (ibid., 70).

In a later book, entitled *Creating Health,* Chopra states:

> The real you is the *arrangement,* the *organizing power,* the *knowledge,* the *intelligence,* the *impulse of consciousness* that designs material stuff to give the appearance of you. That is the only reality worthy to rank as you in your completeness. It is nonmaterial, whole, dynamic, and yet utterly stable, and infinite in its capacity to evolve. (1991, 103)

Chopra's exploration of this model of human beings has led him far from conventional medicine, into the investigation of complementary and alternative treatments now gaining respect in the U.S.

Another major contributor to the cultural acceptance of a unified body and mind has been Candace Pert, the microbiologist with the National Institutes of Health who was able to identify and establish the role of neuropeptides in communicating between cells in the body. According to Pert, these "molecules of emotion" appear everywhere in the body, in trillions of cells, almost simultaneously with whatever stimulus is affecting the emotions. Each emotion has a different set of neuropeptides associated with it, and each set of neuropeptides provides a particular set of instructions to the cells. Even a memory of an event can call forth these chemicals into every part of the body, causing all of our cells to react as if the event were occurring here and now. Her book, *Molecules of Emotion*, firmly established the scientific basis for the effects of thoughts and feelings on the activity of individual cells, throughout the body. and her contribution to the film *What the BLEEP Do We Know!?* has made these ideas accessible to the general public.

On the basis of her research, she concluded that "the subconscious is the body" (Pert 1997), suggesting that all of our memories and deeply held assumptions and beliefs are embedded in the cells and intercellular systems of the body.

Extending Pert's research, Bruce Lipton has been able to describe precisely how the neuropeptides affect the workings of individual cells. In a series of lectures over the past decade, and in his book *Biology of Belief* (2005), Lipton graphically demonstrates the mechanism whereby both the chemical and the electromagnetic signature of chemicals "unlock" the receptors that, in turn, control the chemicals and activities of organelles within the cell. This capacity is the basis for the effectiveness of many modern pharmaceuticals, such as Tamoxifen, which has a molecular "signature" that imitates the structure of estrogen so well that the cell's receptors cannot tell the difference and so accept the inert Tamoxifen molecule, reducing the number of cells affected by the growth-inducing estrogen molecule. Lipton states that matching the electromagnetic signature is enough—whether a chemical is present or not. As a result, he says, the energy of a thought, as much as the chemical structures precipitated by the thought, can change the functioning of a cell.

Mind-Body Evidence: The Placebo Effect

IN *The Future of the Body* (1992), a remarkable compilation of the published research on human development, healing, and consciousness, Michael Murphy points out that "psychophysical changes" are far more common than we normally assume, noting that bodies often "rely on common modalities of change," in "largely dissociated processes." He suggests that "Hysterical stigmata and false pregnancy demonstrate the ... precision with which highly charged images can shape somatic processes," and goes on to state:

> Placebo effects and spiritual healing, too, depend on suggestive imagery, as well as expectation of success, the deliberate or covert practice of healing affirmations, health-mimicking behaviors, and confidence in ... processes. (544)

In his groundbreaking book, *Anatomy of an Illness*, Norman Cousins, the popular former editor of *The Saturday Review,* set forth a theory of medicine that earned him a place on the University of California at Los Angeles Medical School faculty—but is largely ignored by doctors today. Cousins had experienced a serious illness that he was able to overcome through a series of actions that made sense to him but were not recognized as having any significant medical value in themselves. When, upon recovery, he described his self-treatment in an article, more than one noted physician jeeringly ascribed his newfound health to "the placebo effect."

It's interesting to consider this statement in light of the fact that, in tests of a new medication, the goal is always to find out how many more people find relief from their symptoms from the medication than from the "placebo" ("placebo" means "sweet word" and is usually offered in the form of a "sugar pill" or equally ineffective treatment), In fact, in most studies, the "expected" rate of

8

relief from the placebo is 30+ percent: that is, about a third of the people in such tests recover, or have significant reduction in symptoms, simply by taking the placebo. This is even more interesting when one understands the rules of such tests: the new medication must show results that are "significantly higher" than the placebo— where a "significant difference" is typically defined as 1 percent, 5 percent, or 10 percent. This means that a "clinically tested" medication is one that has been demonstrated to show results only slightly higher than the placebo!

Cousins was intrigued by the possibilities and did some research of his own. As documented in his book, he came to the conclusion that "the history of medicine is actually the history of the placebo effect" (1979, 132). Reviewing the "grim array of potions and procedures" medical practitioners have applied to illnesses over the centuries, ranging from using leeches for "bleeding" a patient to placing hot irons on the body, from force-feeding concoctions of herbs and roots to bombarding the body with radiation, he began to see that

> ... people were able to overcome these noxious prescriptions, along with the assorted malaises for which they had been prescribed, because their doctors had given them something far more valuable than the drugs: a robust belief that what they were getting was good for them. They had reached out to their doctors for help; they believed they were going to be helped—and they were. (ibid., 133)

Today, as always, it doesn't take long for healing practitioners to discover that it's not possible to talk about any particular human body without talking about the mind associated with that body. Our thoughts and feelings, our attitudes, and our expectations have all been demonstrated to affect the state of our immune system, our rate of healing, our responses to medications and procedures, and the various cycles and interactions going on within our bodies from moment to moment. So, although the term "psychosomatic" ("psycho" referring to mind and emotions and "somatic" referring to the physiology and anatomy of the body) is often used to discount a set of symptoms as "all in one's head," many medical practitioners—most visibly represented by Deepak Chopra, Larry Dossey, Andrew Weil, and Norman Shealy—have come to accept that virtually every symptom is psychosomatic: a function of the interaction of both mind and body.

Mind-Body Research and Treatment

ONCE THE SPLIT BETWEEN MIND AND BODY was bridged, many lines of inquiry were opened. From anthropologists like Gregory Bateson *(Steps to an Ecology of Mind)* to physicists like Fritjof Capra *(The Tao of Physics)*, Brian Swimme *(The Universe Is a Green Dragon)*, and Bob Toben and Fred Alan Wolfe *(Space-Time and Beyond)*, the scientific literature has proliferated with experiments and theories seeking to unify our experiences of body and mind.

Energy- and Visualization-Based Hands-on Healing

A fascinating line of experimentation began in the late 1950s, when Bernard Grad and his colleagues at McGill University in Canada did a series of tests of the effects of "laying on of hands." In these tests, a self-described "healer" held containers in which mice who were surgically wounded had been placed. The results showed that those mice healed significantly faster and with fewer complications than did the control group. When the same person held containers of water that would be used on barley sprouts, the plants grew taller and stronger than those in control groups. In later experiments, the researchers had other people hold the water containers and found that the plants whose water had been held by people diagnosed with significant psychological problems actually did more poorly than those whose water containers had been held by "healthy" people. These tests and others described by Grad in the *International Journal of Parapsychology* were not well known, but Peter Tompkins and Christopher Bird's book describing similar tests, called *The Secret Life of Plants* (1973), became a best-seller in the 1970s.

During that same decade, Dolores Krieger, professor of nursing at New York University, began to teach and encourage scientific studies of a technique she called Therapeutic Touch (also known as "TT"), which is based on a similar idea. A trained practitioner learns to place a hand on or slightly above a wound or damaged area of the body, learning to "feel" the problem there and "send" healing "energy" to the area. Tens of thousands of people around the world have been taught the technique, many of whom are registered nurses, rigorously trained in the rules and principles of traditional chemical and mechanical Era I medicine. The popularity of TT among nurses is evidence of their belief in the inherent capability to heal and their desire to help people directly, beyond the limits of Era I medical protocol. In clinical trials and many documented cases, TT has been established as a significantly effective tool. As one nurse describes her experience,

> I started practicing TT 15 years ago and used it for a few years before I began to sense energetically. Even now, I don't ... sense many of the things my beginning students do. So why did I keep on practicing? Because I could see that people I worked with were experiencing the relaxation response, pain relief, accelerated wound healing, mental clarity, emotional balance, and/or spiritual connection. (www.therapeutic-touchnetwork.org 1999)

About the same time that Dr. Krieger was introducing Therapeutic Touch to nurses, another hands-on healing method, called *Reiki* (which means "universal life energy" in Japanese) was being introduced from Japan by way of Hawaii. Again, thousands of people have been trained in the technique, many of them licensed massage therapists, with extensive backgrounds in traditional anatomy and physiology. As with TT, *Reiki* practitioners are trained to place a hand on, or slightly above, the body, sense the need, and send healing "energy" into damaged areas. Most have experienced the kind of results described by the nurse, above.

Several randomized, double-blind studies of such "hands-on" healing techniques have been completed, with large numbers of subjects. In the best-known such study, conducted by D. Wirth in 1990, non-contact TT (that is, when the practitioner holds the hands above the body, at the edge of a perceived "field," without actually touching the skin) significantly accelerated the rate of healing for deep skin wounds.

Biofeedback: Demonstration of the Unified Mind-Body

During the late 1960s and early '70s, the idea that the cybernetic learning process of "instant feedback" could be used to assist people dealing with health issues emerged in the popular mind. The Biofeedback Research Society was founded in 1970, and by the mid-1980s thousands of articles on the subject had been published.

Working with the Menninger Foundation in Kansas during the 1970s, Elmer and Alyce Green began to apply these ideas to some common, but difficult-to-treat, health conditions. They set up a series of experiments that let patients observe changes in various recording devices to which they were "hooked up." Many people, children especially, loved the experience of changing the graph on a screen or sheet of paper, generating a tone, or moving a needle on a meter, simply by changing the way they thought or felt. With EEGs, blood-oxygen meters, blood-pressure monitors, stethoscopes, and galvanic skin response (electrodermal activity) meters, the Greens and others taught hundreds of people to adjust their heart rate and rhythm, their circulation, their blood pressure, and even their brain-wave patterns.

It rapidly became clear that, given immediate information about the results of their effort, people could learn to control many normally "involuntary" processes in the body. As they continued their research with other types of scanners and monitors, the Greens concluded, "it may be possible to bring under some degree of voluntary control any physiological process that can continuously be . . . displayed" (Green and Green 1977, 42–43).

In the many tests and experiments that followed, and in practical application, such "biofeedback" (BF) techniques have been used effectively with a wide variety of health conditions. The InteliHealth website lists the following conditions as amenable to BF therapy:

- tension headaches and migraine
- circulatory limitations, such as Raynaud's disease
- digestive disorders, including constipation
- incontinence, both urinary and fecal
- hypertension (high blood pressure)
- cardiac arrhythmias (abnormal heart rhythms)
- addictions
- epilepsy
- sleep disorders
- PMS (premenstrual syndrome)
- ADD, ADHD (attention deficit disorders)
- panic and anxiety disorders

The InteliHealth site also lists several other, more severe conditions related to spinal cord injuries, paralysis, and others, stating that "each year, new illnesses are added to the list of health problems that may respond to biofeedback therapy" (www.InteliHealth.com).

The Mayo Clinic website adds to this list the following:

- asthma
- hot flashes
- nausea and vomiting associated with chemotherapy

The Mayo Clinic site further states that biofeedback therapy "can reduce, or even eliminate, your need for medication … help conditions that have not responded to medication … helps put you in charge of your own healing …" (MayoClinic.com).

In their exhaustive bibliography of Complementary and Alternative Medicine (CAM) Barrows and Jacobs state:

> Children seem to have a particular aptitude and enthusiasm for this therapy. The resemblance that BF shares with video and computer games has been used to great advantage. Also children have less skepticism about this therapy and learn more quickly. (2001, 20)

Children's enthusiasm for BF techniques has led Vincent Monastra of the FPI Attention Disorders Clinic in Endicott, New York, to explore their use with children who were taking Ritalin. Children in his program were given weekly BF training, literally playing a video game with their minds. In these games, the characters moved only when the participant maintained a half-second of activity in the frontal lobe (the region of the brain that is associated with sustained attention and concentration). Monastra found that all of those who participated in the therapy were able to cut their medication by at least half. "… the kids who got biofeedback maintained the gain they achieved with medication, even without the medication" (Kircheimer 2005). Monastra's results are consistent with those of other studies and clinical applications: some therapists have been using biofeedback therapy for ADD and ADHD with consistent success since the '60s.

Murphy (1992) points out that the essential principles of biofeedback are not new. Children have always used various kinds of toys and play to learn motor skills. Anecdotal accounts of individuals controlling their heart rates and muscle responses have been the topic of stories and articles throughout human history. Speech therapists have used various forms of immediate feedback to train those who are hearing- and speech-impaired for nearly a century. The

Mowrers introduced an alarm system triggered by urine to end bedwetting in the 1930s. Others during the same period demonstrated the capacity to learn to totally relax a single muscle. Still, the dominant paradigm of science and medicine has been that there is little, if any, connection between the autonomic nervous system and conscious thought—and few physicians are taught the principles of biofeedback as part of their medical training.

One interesting application of BF techniques has been in the modification of brain-wave patterns. Increased alpha-wave activity, associated with increased overall well-being, has sparked public interest, especially when EEG patterns of experienced *Zen* meditators were shown to have elevated alpha-wave patterns and the public assumed that the "alpha state" and mystical experience were synonymous. However, Murphy's assessment of the research is that there is little connection between the level of alpha-wave activity and the experience of mystical states (1992). Increases in theta, beta, and asymmetrical patterns of multiple wave levels across the hemispheres are other results achieved using BF techniques, along with the increased activity in certain regions noted in the ADD/ADHD studies, above.

Considering the thousands of recorded studies and applications of BF, there is a clear distinction between the results of "BF training" and "BF experiments." When BF is used as a method for training and enhancing the individual's capacity to manage the body, results tend to be much more significant than when BF experiments are set up using "control" and "conditioning" as the ruling parameters. Murphy and the Greens are adamant that the primary utility of biofeedback is self-awareness and self-regulation through volition, resulting in a reduced need for medication.

The Transformative Effects of Imagery

Visualization and guided imagery emerged as a tool with wide-ranging uses in the 1970s. Shakti Gawain's *Creative Visualization*

(1980) was a very popular text through the 1980s, frequently on required reading lists in colleges and universities—even in the usually conservative business schools. A remarkable book by Robert Masters and Jean Houston, called *Mind Games* (1972), provided a guided group process for moving from minimal capacity to visualize to instantaneous achievement of deep-trance states and journeys. By the mid-'80s, both the research and the popular literature were announcing that the process of imagining something fully could have as profound an effect on the mind-body as doing the same activity physically.

The use of visualization as a tool for controlling or eliminating symptoms of disease came into popular awareness in the late 1970s, with the work of Carl Simonton and his cancer support groups. He reported numerous cases in which children and adults were able to reverse tumor growth, relieve pain and pressure, and restore the use of limbs by visualizing processes in the body.

Simonton's experience was that imagery therapy can be an effective medical factor, recognizing that the patient's healing intention is essential to its success. It communicates with the mind-body from the inside to help heal. From the beginning of the development of imagery therapy, the mind-body effect accessed nonordinary realities. The source of power of the imagery used depends on the patient and on transpersonal factors beyond ordinary consciousness. He encouraged the use of meaningful symbols as much as possible, so, for many of his patients, white blood cells became soldiers, fighting off the alien hordes, or they were tiny bulldozers carving out the mountain of the tumor and hauling away their loads; for others, the bone marrow became factories, producing healthy blood cells of all types, or the blood vessels became rivers, flowing toxins out to the "port" of the kidneys and bladder.

In this process, one relaxes the body to elevate the alpha-wave activity of the brain and allow an internal experience of visual, auditory, and other sense-related images—drawn initially from memory and imagination. As Jeanne Achterberg put it,

… messages have to undergo translation by the right hemisphere into nonverbal or imagerial terminology before they can be understood by the involuntary or autonomic nervous system…. imagery … is the medium of communicating between consciousness and the internal environment of our bodies … (1985, 123–24)

Visual symbols are rendered more effective by the emotional "load" they carry.

Frank Lawlis, a psychiatrist using imagery and other approaches in his pain clinic, found visualization processes particularly helpful in working with his patients and found support for his experience in the research literature:

… the research evidence continues to grow, showing that a patient's imaging can have a positive influence on the healing process in such conditions as pruritic eczema, acne *vulgaris*, birth pain, diabetes, breast cancer, arthritis, migraine and tension headaches, and treatment of severe burns. (1996, 115)

Part of Lawlis' success lay in the fact that he didn't insist on "visualization" but, rather, worked with the whole range of senses, building on the faculty of eidetic imagery. Visual imagination has great potential, but so does auditory imagination. Some people feel limited with visual imagination but may make important use of audio-guidance. Imagery therapy may soon develop methods that access inner senses of people who have limitations in visual-imaginal or auditory-imaginal therapies. Imagery medicine will probably discover new ways to work with imagination and mind in mind-body medicine.

This expansion from the strictly visual to the other senses has the effect, as Masters and Houston (1972) point out, of engaging the full mind-body system in the process.

The most powerful imagery for people suffering from chronic pain is kinesthetic in nature ... dependent on proprioceptive faculties of our bodymind ... the pleasure we derive from dancing or playing a sport.... asking patients to feel their heart relaxing, slowing down, radiating warmth out to their hands and feet as they picture themselves moving slowly around a warm, crackling campfire on a summer beach ... and the blood pressure normalizes. (109)

The more senses that are engaged, the more effective the process is in persuading the mind-body that the experience is "real." Vividly imagined experiences, including odors, sensations, felt-movements, sounds, and tastes, as well as colors, depth, and emotional responses, are, according to Masters and Houston and other researchers, the most effective, by far.

Transpersonal Studies

THE FIELD OF TRANSPERSONAL STUDIES emerged in this country as a result of the human potential movement of the 1960s. Formally, the Association for Transpersonal Psychology (ATP) split off from the Association for Humanistic Psychology in the early 1970s, as an increasing number of scholars from many disciplines began to explore and explain various cultural phenomena, personal experiences, and spiritual traditions that seemed to transcend the mind-body model of the human being that was dominant in that period.

As Lawlis put it, transpersonal psychology "depicts evolutionary growth as coming from *beyond the self*, as a power larger or bigger than the individual ... The basic tenet of this approach is that the destiny of humanity is the evolution of the human spirit ..." (1996, xvi).

Transpersonal psychology is both a practice and a field of research. As a practice, transpersonal therapists

... assume within each individual planes of wisdom beyond the primary intellectual strength of the ego. They use therapeutic strategies that attempt to bring out from inner sources the knowledge of the unconscious.... [The transpersonal therapist] views healing as the result of harmonizing and balancing the body-mind-spirit dynamics within a person's sphere of being.... It sees fellowship with others—community—as one of the strongest influences on our own transformational potential ... (Lawlis 1996, xvii)

Among the disciplines contributing to this relatively new field of study are: anthropology, psychology, communications studies and cybernetics, religious studies, and consciousness research. The major focus of the research has been understanding the ways that human experience is affected by external influences that have not been measurable by physical means. Thus, distance healing, meditation, shamanic practices, and the "group consciousness" of organizations and communities have been typical topics at conferences and in journals. Roger Walsh, Frances Vaughan, Joanna Macy, and Angeles Arrien are among the best-known names in this field, through their books describing the models and processes of many cultures and therapies that contribute to the field.

During the same years that ATP was coming into existence, astronaut Edgar Mitchell returned from his journeys in space determined to understand more fully the nature of consciousness. With the support of friends and colleagues, he launched the Institute of Noetic Sciences (IONS). The mission of IONS is to facilitate and communicate scientific research regarding the previously discounted and misunderstood experiences called, variously, "mystical," "psychic," and "spiritual." In 1976, Willis Harman, a retired engineering professor who created the futures studies groups at Stanford Research Institute, was appointed director of IONS. Under his leadership the Institute was established as a major contributor to understanding such phenomena in both the scientific and lay communities. The

Institute's current journal, *Shift,* outlines research priorities and results and offers readers a variety of opportunities to experience and test the ideas that IONS is exploring. IONS has engaged in a number of intriguing research projects on its own, including, among many others:

A study on distant healing intention to help late-stage AIDS patients, published in the *Western Journal of Medicine.*

A study on the possible effects of Qi Gong on brain-tumor cells in a state-of-the-art laboratory setting that continues under the sponsorship of the National Institutes of Health.

A study comparing a distant healing vs. control group (no distant healing) with a placebo group on acceleration of wound healing in women with breast cancer by Marilyn Schlitz, PhD, Harriett Hopf, MD, and Cassandra Vieten, PhD.

A study of the physiological synchronization between healer and patient involved the development and use of neurophysiological techniques to evaluate hypotheses emerging from the field of mind-body medicine by Leanna Standish, PhD, Deepak Chopra, MD, and Marilyn Schlitz, PhD.

A study researching the impact of external Qi Gong on cancer cells: effects of dose and distance, testing the hypothesis that human gene expression responds to the effects of intentionality on the part of Qi Gong masters operating from a distance, by Garret Yount, PhD, and Chinese Academy of Medical Sciences, Beijing, China.

The rigorously scientific approach taken in these studies has done much to bring the potential of transpersonal experience into the realm of Western scientific medicine.

Traditional Mind-Body Medicine

ALTHOUGH WE HAVE SEEN increasing popularity of methods like acupuncture, homeopathy, massage, and herbs as healing methods in the U.S. and Europe, these have been typically portrayed by the medical establishment as methods for minimizing symptoms by enhancing the patient's comfort. Their use as therapies in the context of a unified mind-body is limited to a few practitioners scattered across the continents.

One possible exception is the very recent interest in an energy-based healing method from China called *Chi Gung, Ki Gung,* or, sometimes, *Qi Gong.* In this method, which is closely related to the more familiar *Tai Chi Chuan,* one moves one's body in ways that facilitate energy movement while visualizing the energy entering, moving through, and supporting organs or tissues that are weak or diseased. The movement provides a kinesthetic, as well as visual, focus for imagery—and also a means for immediate feedback from the body as energy flows are visualized and felt. This integration of several modalities in one method has proved powerful for many of its practitioners—both for healing and for maintaining a sense of well-being. The remarkable results from the use of this method have been documented by many researchers and made popular by Gregg Braden in his popular book, *The Isaiah Effect.*

An entirely different approach comes from the shamanic traditions of indigenous cultures around the world. From these, we get the use of many herbs and potions, but we also get the use of crystals in healing, with different gemstones being related to different conditions and symptoms, based on their color and crystalline form. The theory for crystal healing is straightforward: the body is predominantly energetic in nature and crystals resonate with different energy patterns (note, for example, the old "crystal radios" built in the early twentieth century by running an electric current through a piece of quartz to get sounds from radio waves). As the body and crystal come into contact, the resonant pattern of the crystal and the pattern of the energetic movement in the area around the crystal move into alignment, bringing a reduction or elimination of any symptoms resulting from the disharmonious "vibrations." In addition, certain crystals have the capacity for "storing" vibratory patterns that the shaman may "bless" or "empower" them with, thus enhancing their capacity for restoring balance wherever they are placed.

Shamanic healers also use rhythmic music and movement in their healing practices for similar reasons. In addition, they set up rituals to relieve anxiety and stress, encouraging the patient to relax and release normal patterns of thought. Some shamanic traditions include laying on of hands, as well. And virtually all shamanic traditions include the practice of visualization as a means for gaining insight into, and power over, the condition being experienced.

The idea of a unified mind-body system as a basis for medical treatment is by no means established within Western scientific and medical circles. It is, however, well founded in both experience and laboratory experiments—which both suggest and call for a new model of the human being, one that explains these research results and offers new possibilities for treatment.

References

Achterberg, Jeanne. *Imagery in Healing*. Boston: Shambhala, 1985.

Barrows, Kevin A., and Bradly P. Jacobs. "Mind-Body Medicine: An Introduction and Review of the Literature," draft, September 2001.

Bateson, Gregory. *Steps Toward an Ecology of Mind*. New York: Ballantine, 1975.

"Biofeedback." www.InteliHealth.com, June 2005.

"Biofeedback: Using the Power of Your Mind to Improve Your Health." MayoClinic.com, June 2005.

Braden, Gregg. *The Isaiah Effect*. New York: Three Rivers Press, 2000.

Chopra, Deepak. *Creating Health*. New York: Houghton-Mifflin, 1991.

———. *Quantum Healing*. New York: Bantam, 1990.

Cousins, Norman. *Anatomy of an Illness from a Patient's Perspective*. New York: Norton, 1979.

Eliade, Mircea. *Shamanism*. Princeton, NJ: Princeton University Press, 1964.

Gawain, Shakti. *Creative Visualization*. San Rafael, CA: New World Library, 1980.

Green, Elmer, and Alyce Green. *Beyond Biofeedback*. New York: Dell, 1977.

Kircheimer, Sid. "Biofeedback Enhances ADHD Treatments." WebMD.com, June 2005.

Lawlis, G. Frank. *Transpersonal Medicine*. Boston: Shambhala, 1996.

Lipton, Bruce. *Biology of Belief*. Santa Rosa, CA: Elite Books, 2005.

Masters, Robert, and Jean Houston. *Mind Games*. New York: Delta, 1972.

Miller, Iona, and Richard Miller. "Biophysics / Mindbody." nexus-magazine.com, 2004.

Murphy, Michael. *The Future of the Body: Explorations into the Further Evolution of Human Nature*. Los Angeles: Tarcher, 1992.

Pert, Candace. *Molecules of Emotion*. New York: Touchstone, 1997.

Toben, Bob, and Fred Alan Wolfe. *Space-Time and Beyond*. New York: Bantam, 1983.

Tompkins, Peter, and Christopher Bird. *The Secret Life of Plants*. New York: HarperCollins, 1973.

Wirth, D. 1990. "The Effect of Non-Contact Therapeutic Touch on the Healing of Full Thickness Dermal Wounds." *Subtle Energies* 1 (1990): 1–20.

CHAPTER 2

Meditation Methods Across Cultures

Shamanic Traditions

THE SHAMANIC TRADITIONS HAVE GROWN out of an ancient set of practices, deeply rooted in all Earth-centered cultures. These are the practices of the wise ones, those who have separated themselves from the normal life of village or tribe to master their own emotions and physical responses and to develop the capacity to expand their awareness beyond their bodies and use their will for the good of their communities.

The men and women who have been so singled out are called "shamans" by anthropologists, because the first well-documented experience of these practices was in a Siberian tribe that called such a practitioner *saman.* Shamans use a variety of disciplines to accomplish their goals, and many of their practices continue today, both in the "primitive" tribes of out-of-the-way places and in the "civilized" religious rites of both Eastern and Western traditions.

Michael Harner's *The Way of the Shaman* (1991)—both the book and the follow-up workshops and trainings—brought the essential concepts of shamanic traditions into Western culture. Doing so, he provided a context for such previously popular writings as those of Carlos Castaneda and Lynn Andrews. Since then, numerous books have been printed and studies completed exploring the nature and effectiveness of shamanic practices.

However, Mircea Eliade's *Shamanism: Archaic Techniques of Ecstasy* (1964) remains the classic synthesis of the anthropological literature on the subject. Looking across cultures, he saw consistent patterns: trance states in which the soul was believed to leave the body and travel to other worlds, often by means of a ladder or staircase, and the use of secret languages, taught by spirits who travel on the ladder. These elements, he suggested, may contribute to the effectiveness of shamans as healers and prophets in their communities.

The fact that there are certain consistencies across cultures, in both principles and practice, should not be too surprising, because some things simply work, wherever they are applied. Among the practices common across shamanic traditions are the following:

- turning off "normal" thought processes to become silent inside, then to listen to the body and the environment

- disciplines to learn to manage the sensations of the body

- study of the culture's traditions that explain how the world works and how people's minds, bodies, and communities function and develop

- study of one's own thought processes, dreams, and imaginations

- specific movements and sounds to enhance awareness, physical strength and agility, and overall well-being

- use of various movements, chemicals, mental discipline, and other methods for achieving altered states of consciousness in which awareness moves beyond the range of normal senses, space, and time

These practices may be found among the Maori of New Zealand and the Eskimos of Alaska, among the hill tribes of Southeast Asia and the "witches" of Bulgaria, among the indigenous tribes of North America and those of the Amazon and Congo. They are also found in Buddhist, Taoist, and Hindu temple communities and in mystical Christian, Muslim, and Jewish communities; and they are the essence of the Sufi tradition.

Each culture has its own specific training protocols, disciplines, and expectations for these practices. Each culture has particular understandings of the nature of the shamanic experience, based on that culture's understanding of the nature of the world. Fundamentally, however, they achieve the same end: the enhancement of the individual's capacity to "see" the world in terms of the energy patterns that compose our material experience, to "hear" thoughts and sound patterns that affect the individual and community seeking assistance, to act on the body-mind system of individuals in the community in a way that restores balance and harmony to the individual and the community as a whole, and to perceive outside of normal space and time to forecast or prophesy important shifts and changes that affect the well-being of the community.

Judeo-Christian Mystic Traditions

CHRISTIANITY IS LARGELY BASED on the capacity of one person, called Jesus, to heal others through touch and the spoken word—and his directive to his disciples to go out and do the same. Descriptions of the early churches—both in the Bible and from other sources—always include people healing each other through prayer and laying on of hands. The apostle to the Gentiles, Paul, includes healing and prophesying among the gifts of the Spirit that come with becoming a Christian, and gives some guidelines for developing the capacity to do so. Peter, John, and the others are reported by Luke to have effected healings when their shadows crossed sick people laid out along the streets where they walked.

The expectation of healing as part of being Christian was lost to the public and church congregations for centuries, until the emergence of "sacred relics" as vehicles for miraculous powers in the

Middle Ages. From the eleventh century forward, pious Christians could go to a chapel or cathedral and touch, or simply view, a bit of bone or cloth they believed to be associated with a saint or holy person, and often feel whatever pain or symptom that had troubled them fall away. The belief and expectation were enhanced by the presence of crutches, bandages, slings, and other prosthetic devices left behind by those who went away healed. It's only in well-attended shrines, often little-known outside their area, that are scattered across the planet that this tradition remains alive today.

In convents and monasteries, however, the expectation of the miraculous remained alive well into the twentieth century. Stories of nuns and monks in ecstatic trance, levitating, healing others through prayer or touch, living only on water or on the communion offered at daily Mass, and seeing profoundly moving visions of Jesus, his mother, and various saints, have circulated throughout the cloistered orders for centuries—and still do.

A famous recent set of stories concerns an Italian monk, Padre Pio. Many anecdotes describing his capacities are told, ranging from his stigmata to his levitations, many of which have been documented. Caroline Myss tells of World War II pilots, sent to bomb an Italian village, turning back because a monk seemed to be floating in the air above it, indicating that they should go elsewhere— while witnesses in the monastery below observed the good monk praying in his cell that God would protect the village.

These stories, and the new interest in the Bible made possible by the reforms of the Vatican II Council of Bishops, inspired the birth of the charismatic movement within the Catholic Church during the 1960s and '70s. This movement, similar in many ways to American Pentecostalism, has since expanded into mainstream Protestantism, where it has met the Pentecostal revivalist traditions of ecstatic trances and "faith healing." Priests such as Ron Roth have found themselves, like Pentecostal ministers, touching people or speaking a few words and watching the infirm get up and walk away (Roth 2000). These clerics have felt what they call the

Holy Spirit guiding them to say things and do things in church services that have led to the remission of cancers and other "terminal" illnesses among members of their congregations. And many of their experiences have been thoroughly documented using the scientific method.

Yet such miracles are not confined to Christian monks and mystics. Jesus was, after all, a Nazarene, dedicated to God in the Temple at Jerusalem and preaching in the synagogues around Judea and Galilee, as well as in the Temple itself. His healing miracles, the Jewish Talmud and other histories of the period tell us, were hardly unique. Many wandering preachers performed similar healings — perhaps best known of whom was Simon Magus who, in the years following Jesus' crucifixion, traveled to Rome and performed many similar miracles there. And a cursory look at the Old Testament, particularly the stories of Elijah and Elisha, makes it clear that healing the sick, raising the dead, and prophesying the consequences of current actions were an expectation of one who had dedicated himself to God.

In modern Judaism, these kinds of experiences become possible for those who study the *Qabalah*, the mystery tradition based on a map of consciousness called The Tree of Life. It involves complex numerology and other symbology as means of focusing attention, stilling the mind of its normal thought patterns, and allowing the perception of a "still small voice," that of *Shekinah*, the wisdom that is the feminine aspect of the divinity. Having accomplished this, the practitioner becomes empowered — as a healer and a prophet, for the good of his family and his community.

> There are many ways of using the *Qabalah* for healing. . . . The Tree of Life, being a map of the whole person, is an ideal model to use for healing, whether of ourselves or others. A "whole healing" of any individual will include the whole Tree of Life — body, personality, soul and Spirit. For the healing to be effective it will also include the relationship of the individual with their external world . . . on many levels, from

the physical, through the psychological, to the deepest levels of spiritual connection ...

... using the Tree as a healer of energy disorders and imbalances ... it is undoubtedly true that we need to be clear vessels for the reception and transmission of the energies engendered by such work. (Parfitt 1994, 101ff.)

Another tradition deriving from Judeo-Christian roots was originally called Christian Science and has since split into two groups: the Church of Christ, Scientist, commonly called Christian Science, and the various churches that make up what is known as the New Thought movement—including Unity, Religious Science, Divine Science, and the Church of Truth.

These two groups emerged from the work of Ralph Waldo Emerson and a healer in mid-nineteenth-century Maine named Phineas Parkhurst Quimby who believed he had discovered the method used by Jesus Christ and felt that it was possible for anyone to learn the process. One of his patients, a homeopathic physician named Mary Baker Patterson, studied with Quimby and then, following his death, developed her own version of his methods and described them in her classic work, *Science and Health with Key to the Scriptures*. Having used these methods for her own healing, Mrs. Patterson traveled around New England, offering her healing services. In 1875 she settled in Lynn, Massachusetts, where she set up a small school to teach them. There she married a man named Asa Eddy, and with him founded what is known as the Christian Science Church in Boston and rapidly accrued thousands of members, building the grand "Mother Church," now a major Boston landmark. Perhaps the most famous of Mrs. Eddy's accomplishments is the creation of the still-functioning international newspaper, *The Christian Science Monitor*. Perhaps the best known of her disciples has been Joel Goldsmith, who was a world-famous healer and teacher in the mid-twentieth century and went on to found The Infinite Way.

One of Mrs. Eddy's students, Emma Curtis Hopkins, a high school teacher with a lifelong interest in classical philosophy, found Mrs. Eddy's system to be limited and not entirely coherent. So, when she set up her own school in Chicago, she offered a slightly different version of the methods, now published in the text *Scientific Christian Mental Practice*. She healed hundreds and trained thousands of people, including the founders of Unity, Church of Truth, and Divine Science. Then she closed the school and worked individually. In her last years, she taught Ernest Holmes, the founder of Religious Science. Students of her students include Emmet Fox, Catherine Ponder, Florence Scovel Shinn, and James Dillet Freeman, to name a few of the better-known New Thought teachers and writers.

These traditions have several things in common, based on their originators' experiences with healing and maintaining health and prosperity.

- They assume that illness and poverty are products of the workings of one's thoughts and feelings.

- They offer a 12-step process for developing the capacity to change the mind's normal processes, replacing "old thoughts" with a "New Thought."

- They encourage the negation and release of thoughts and ideas that lead to illness and the affirmation of thoughts and ideas that support health and well-being.

- They accept the possibility that one person can affect the mind-body of another, and they emphasize the need to frequently go within to discover a deeper Truth or Reality in any situation.[5]

---

5. This "going within" process is very similar to the meditation techniques taught to the Fillmores by Yogananda in Unity and is like prayer in Christian Science.

The traditions differ in some basic assumptions about the nature of the body and of divinity, and in the emphasis in the Christian Science church on Mrs. Eddy's revelation as the only source of understanding (Miller 2000).

The Science of Mind, written by Ernest Holmes in 1925, following his series of lessons with Mrs. Hopkins, is perhaps the best-known work describing the essence of New Thought principles and practices. In it, he states:

> Through spiritual discernment, we see that we have within us a power which is greater than anything we shall ever contact; a power that can overcome every obstacle in our experience and set us safe, satisfied, and at peace, healed and prosperous in a new light and a new life … The storehouse of nature is filled with infinite good, awaiting the touch of our awakened thought to spring forth into manifestation in our lives … The word that we speak is the law of our lives, and nothing hinders its operation but ourselves. (1998, 146)

Today, millions of people around the world use these basic principles and rely on the services of thousands of teachers and practitioners from these churches, with many documented healings—of body, mind, economy, and relationships—occurring each year in each church.

Yoga: Well-Being Through Union

MUCH OF THE EARLY RESEARCH on meditation and its effects involved *yogis* from India. Westerners have long been fascinated by the range of skills and capacities demonstrated by long-term practitioners of this ancient science. Reports of remarkable feats of control over the body, coupled with the sometimes overwhelming charisma of the more famous masters, fueled curiosity and concern. While most Westerners think of the postures associated with *hatha yoga*, there are at least eight different *yogas*, each focusing on a different aspect of human development. Some of these are: *bhakti yoga*, the path of devotion; *prana yoga*, the mastery of energy flows through the breath; *karma yoga*, the path of action in the world; *raja yoga*, mastery of the whole self through the path of reason and intellect; and *tantra yoga*, mastery of the body through disciplined sensory experience. Each of these disciplines has been followed and taught by students and masters for millennia. Each of them has a whole unique set of principles and practices—and several different "schools" or approaches, with variations on those principles and practices—taught by different lineages of teachers.

It would be fair to say that the several *yogas* are prehistoric practices, handed down through generations of priests and teachers in the *Vedic* traditions that are now known, collectively, as Hinduism. References to these practices may be found in the oldest known religious texts, called the *Vedas*, written in the root Indo-European language, Sanskrit, some 5,000 years ago. Many of the fundamental principles may be found in one small portion of those manuscripts, a sacred Hindu text called the *Bhagavad Gita*.[6] It is the story of a young man's encounter with divinity—in the form of Krishna (sometimes called the Hindu Christ)—and the many lessons that divine being imparts to him.

The ancient word *yoga* is commonly translated as "union" and is the root of the English word "yoke." It is defined in the *Gita* as "the breaking of contact with pain." In practice, *yoga* is a path—often described as a shortcut—to the continuous experience of non-local, nonattached awareness, or liberation, called, in Sanskrit, *moksha*, or *samadhi*. "The Atman [Real Self] shines forth in its own pristine nature, as pure consciousness" (Isherwood and Prabhavananda 1953, 221). All the practice, all the principles, and all the

---

6. Made famous in the West by Gandhi's devotion to its precepts and disciplined study of the text, the *Gita* is one of the most widely read books in the world and is available in a number of English translations.

variations of *yoga* are designed to achieve this one end.

Along the way, *yoga* practices help the practitioner be healthier, happier, and more effective. Section One of the ancient *Yoga Sutras of Patanjali* includes the following aphorisms:

> 30. Sickness, mental laziness, doubt, lack of enthusiasm, sloth, craving for sense-pleasure, false perception, despair caused by failure to concentrate and unsteadiness in concentration: these distractions are the obstacles to knowledge.
>
> 31. These distractions are accompanied by grief, despondency, trembling of the body and irregular breathing.
>
> 32. They can be removed by the practice of concentration upon a single truth.
>
> (ibid., 64–66)

The translators go on to say, "In order to achieve this concentration, we must calm and purify our minds" (ibid., 66), which, Patanjali tells us, may be done by changing our attitudes toward the people and events around us, and "The mind may also be calmed by [breathing] *prana*" (ibid., 68).

Because of the enhanced capacities that come with the concentration required in the practices of the various *yogas*, many practitioners find themselves experiencing what, in our culture, are often called "paranormal" or "psychic" events. Patanjali says, in Section Three of his aphorisms, that, through such concentration, the mind:

> ... passes beyond the three kinds of changes which take place in subtle or gross matter and in the organs: change of form, change of time, and change of condition.... one obtains knowledge of the past and the future ... of what is subtle, hidden, and distant ... of the constitution of the body....
> [O]ne gains mastery of the elements ... also perfection of the body, which is no longer subject to the obstructions of the elements ... one gains mastery of the organs ... (ibid., 182ff.)

One of the best-known *yoga* practices in this country is the *kriya yoga* brought to the U.S. in the 1920s by Paramahansa Yogananda, founder of the Self-Realization Fellowship (Yogananda 1946). He describes his method as follows:

> *Kriya Yoga* is a simple, psychophysiological method by which human blood is decarbonated and recharged with oxygen. The atoms of this extra oxygen are transmuted into life-current to rejuvenate the brain and spinal centers. By stopping the accumulation of veinous blood, the *yogi* is able to lessen or prevent the decay of tissues. The advanced *yogi* transmutes his cells into energy ... uses his technique to saturate and feed his physical cells with undecayable light ... (ibid., 275ff.)

The earliest documented observations of meditation were with *yogis* in India in the late 1800s. Since then, accomplished masters have been buried for hours and days at a time without harm, monitored through a variety of seemingly impossible tasks, and observed closely by biologists, anthropologists, sociologists, and psychologists (Murphy 1992, 464ff.; Chopra 1987). As the most ancient documented set of mind-body practices, the *yogas* may be considered the first mind-body science. They provide the disciplined practitioner with the capacity to manage sensation, expand sensation beyond the body, overcome desire and attachment, along with the physical and emotional consequences of same, and exert influence on other objects and events. They have been proved over and over, both within India and in Western scientific tradition.

Ayurveda

ONE OF THE MANY GIFTS Deepak Chopra has brought to Western interest in healing is the native Indian system of healing known as *Ayurveda* (*Ayur* referring to "life" and *veda* meaning "science"). In all of his books, and at his healing centers in Lancaster,

Massachusetts, and San Diego, California, Chopra has shown Westerners how healing can be accelerated through the combinations of diet, supplements, activity, meditation, and sound that make up the *Ayurvedic* approach. Though most Americans focus on the diet and supplements, Chopra emphasizes the role of meditation and sound in the practice. In *Quantum Healing* he describes their role and potential.

> In Ayurveda, bliss is the basis for three extremely powerful healing techniques. The first is meditation ... Its importance is that it takes the mind out of its boundaries and exposes it to an unbounded state of consciousness. The other two ... are ... the Ayurvedic psycho-physiological technique ... (we often prefer to use an informal name, the bliss technique) ... [and] ... primordial sound....
>
> The bliss technique gives the patient the experience of himself as pure awareness, the ocean of well-being that is our basic prop and sustenance. With this technique alone it is possible to "drown" a disease in awareness and cure it....
>
> [T]o focus attention more precisely to heal ... the primordial sound technique exists.... With it, a specific tumor or arthritic joint can be attended to; a weak heart of clogged arteries can be zeroed in on. You are not attacking the disorder with the primordial sound but paying closer attention to it—so close that the distortion of awareness lurking at the bottom of the disorder falls back into line....
>
> In Ayurveda, each and every symptom of disease, from a minor neck pain to a full-blown cancer, is under the control of attention.... The Ayurvedic approach is to take a process already going on in the body and assist it naturally and without strain.... Assuming that you are normally constituted, there is no innate reason why you cannot heal any disease with awareness. (1990, 237–39)

In this focus on awareness, *Ayurveda* relies on and embraces the *yoga* traditions of the Hindu culture in which it has emerged.

At the same time, with arrival of Tibetan masters, Buddhist *yogas*[7] have been brought into Western cultures, adding to the rich treasure-chest of ancient methods available to us with significant transformative potential.

Tibetan Wisdom

IT'S PROBABLE THAT NO NATION in the twentieth century was more completely destroyed than Tibet, and yet, marvelously, probably no nation has been able to give more to the expanding paradigm of human life. The reason is twofold. When China crushed defenseless Tibet in 1958 and 1959, there was a tragic mass exodus of the Tibetan people through the Himalayas into India, a dangerous exodus in which the Tibetans were hunted by the Chinese army and often overwhelmed by severe weather. It is estimated that only one out of 100 people succeeded in reaching India to survive, while many died of starvation and exhaustion in the process. But remarkably many of Tibet's greatest living Buddhist masters and doctors survived, protected by the people they led toward survival. These great men carried into India and then into the West profound knowledge of human psychology and potential, and systems of training, kept alive for humanity for centuries in their remote mountain monasteries and villages.

Tibet has so much to offer to the world because of events beginning in the first half of the seventh century, during the time of King Srongtsan Gampo. Tibet was then beginning a reign as a major power in Central Asia that was to last some 200 years. All around

---

7. Because Buddhism grew out of Hinduism many Hindu terms and practices have been maintained within the Buddhist tradition—even as some Judaic practices remain in Christianity and Islam.

Tibet were Buddhist nations—India, China, Nepal, Afghanistan, and Kashmir—in which the Buddhist teachings were flourishing. Srongtsan Gampo converted to Buddhism and began to bring Buddhist books into Tibet. There had been no written Tibetan language. One was derived from Sanskrit, which made possible accurate translations from Sanskrit and Pali. Srongtsan Gampo also sought to strengthen Tibet's medical knowledge.

"In pursuit of medical knowledge, the king held the first international medical conference in Tibet. Doctors came from India, Persia, and China" (Clifford, 1984, 53). Each of the doctors translated one of their essential medical texts into Tibetan. The Persian medical system incorporated the ancient Greek medical system, the basis of Western medicine. "The visiting Persian doctor, Galenos, was asked to remain in Tibet as the court physician. He married and had three sons, all of whom began separate medical family lineages" (ibid). Thus ancient Western medical knowledge had a living lineage in Tibet.

Then, during the reign of King Trisong Detsun, there was a major development in the history of Tibetan knowledge. The king was inspired to further increase the presence of the Buddhist teachings in Tibet. In 749 he sent envoys to invite Padmasambhava, a widely renowned Buddhist master, to bring Buddhist wisdom and power into Tibet. There had been obstructions to the implementation of Buddhism in Tibet. Padmasambhava, called "The Second Buddha" by the Tibetans, knew that the envoys were coming to find him. In his homeland of Uddiyana, presently Afghanistan, where the *Vajrayana* Buddhist teachings had arisen, and in Ghandhara, south of Uddiyana, once a great center of Buddhism, there had been devastation by invading barbarian Huns. Thousands of Buddhist shrines, monasteries, and temples had been desecrated by the seventh century. Padmasambhava saw that the Buddhist teachings and much of ancient wisdom, including profound medical knowledge, could be preserved in Tibet for the future.

What happened subsequently is one of the great events of human history and is remarkably well documented (Yeshe Tsogyal, 1993; Dudjom Rinpoche, 1991).[8] The combination of Padmasambhava's spiritual power and King Trisong Detsun's royal power and grace was able to bring into Tibet not only essential collections of Buddhist scriptures from all Buddhist schools, but the texts and living embodiments of almost all of ancient wisdom, including medicine, astrology, white mathematics, and other revered ancient sciences. In Buddhism, spiritual knowledge and medical knowledge were and are considered inseparable. At that time Tibet was able to bring in sacred texts of Ayurvedic medicine and doctors who embodied that knowledge; revered texts of Chinese medicine and doctors who embodied that knowledge; and medical wisdom of Kashmir, Mongolia, Nepal, Sinkiang, Afghanistan, and Persia.

For more than twenty years an incomparable field of operations was assembled to translate and transmit ancient wisdom. The finest young Tibetans were selected and trained to be translators, some of them sent to countries abroad to learn the languages of the texts being translated. The translations were so carefully made that today some of them are being translated back into their original languages (Clifford, 1984, 56). "By the thirteenth century the Moslems had swept over the Indian regions and utterly destroyed all traces of Buddhist religion, culture, and learning ... This meant two things: first, Tibetans could no longer go to India for teachings, but this was not so important since they had already brought almost all spiritual and scientific lineages back to Tibet as living initiated lineages" (ibid, 58).

The assembled treasury of Tibetan knowledge became the basis for training in medicine as well as in the meditation sciences—a system of training that lasted into the twentieth century. Then,

---

8. A bibliography with reference to Tibetan history, psychology, and medicine is presented in the back of this book. We encourage people to read at least Yeshe Tsogyal's *The Lotus-Born*, her record of the life of Padmasambhava and the events that followed his arrival in Tibet.

because of the Chinese invasion, this system was forced to come out of Tibet and into the world, in the Tibetan diaspora. From the 1960s onward, Tibetan Buddhist teachers and doctors came into the Cold War era, with its vast nuclear arsenals, and the associated stresses of the Age of Anxiety.

Considering briefly the complexity of Tibetan medicine, we can identify three levels.

The first level, traditional Tibetan medicine, is based on Chinese, *Ayurvedic,* and other medical systems brought into Tibet in the seventh and eighth centuries but has its own distinctive characteristics. With the basic requirement of a compassionate nature and a good intelligence, through a training of more than ten years, the student learned the medicinal properties of thousands of plants and various other natural substances selected and compounded to produce sophisticated medicines, acquiring knowledge of the short- and long-term effects of the medicines. Training in human psychological nature and its relation to disease conditions was essential, giving a strong basis of diagnosis as well as treatment. Medical capabilities included surgery, childbirth, near-death care, and after-death care.

The second level of Tibetan medicine could be said to be represented by doctors who were also highly trained lamas, or meditation masters. Dr. Trogawa Rinpoche, who has visited the West several times since 1982, represents this level. In accordance with Buddhist tradition, he was highly regarded in his past incarnation as both a doctor and an incarnate lama, a consciously reincarnated spiritual teacher of the highest order, who carried profound spiritual/psychological, as well as medical, knowledge. He brought great experience into this life, incarnating as Trogawa Rinpoche, and was trained, from the youngest age, to bring that human endowment to an even higher level of capability and realization.

The third level of Tibetan medicine can be partly understood thanks to publications such as Tulku Thondrup's *Hidden Treasures of Tibet* (1986), disclosing the multidimentional nature of *terma,* "hidden treasure." These rare forms of knowledge were concealed by

Padmasambhava in the eighth century, in the unconditioned minds of his close disciples, in the earth, and in works of art.

The subsequent discovery of many of these hidden treasures and the utilization of their transmissions are described in Thondrup's book. However, the nature and utilization of medical *termas* is rarely disclosed, only through direct transmission, and so is unpublished. At this time we can say that Padmasambhava saw unobstructedly and compassionately into the future, and saw the psychological and medical problems of our age.

In the eighth century Yeshe Tsogyal recorded Padmasambhava's revelations in which he defined more than 350 disease conditions of our age that would be mostly undiagnosed or wrongly diagnosed. Some of his medical *termas* contain explicit instructions for psychological and medical treatments of AIDS and other conditions. A few surviving Tibetan lamas, such as Shenphen Dawa Rinpoche, son and lineage heir of the legendary lama Dudjom Rinpoche, are believed to be reincarnated *tertons* and doctors and have knowledge of how to utilize medical *termas*. How fully such knowledge will be utilized, preserved, developed, and passed on to future generations remains to be seen.

The vast and growing potential of Buddhist psychological methods and knowledge of the basis of disease conditions is well documented by now. When Buddhist scriptures and transmission systems were brought up into Tibet in the eighth century, the work was comprehensive and profound. The scriptures and transmissions of all Buddhist schools were included, systems of meditation science that had been developed over a 1,500-year history. The Buddha presented a great science of human development. He taught on ordinary and nonordinary levels for fifty years and revealed three distinct stages of evolutionary training, encompassing the three major Buddhist schools that were to evolve: *Hinayana, Mahayana,* and *Vajrayana.*

The *Vajrayana* Buddhism of Tibet includes the *Hinayana* and *Mahayana* teachings and transmissions and may be the most complete system of human development available on our planet. It is characterized by a range of methods appropriate for the whole spectrum of human psychological types and levels. It offers a sophisticated sense of human problems and the basis of disease conditions, as well as the potentials obstructed by those reductive problems and conditions. For the purpose of this book we are going to focus on three methods that may have important health care impacts in the expanding medical paradigm:

- *Vipashyana* (*Lha Tong* in Tibetan); "mindfulness meditation"
- Vase Breathing (*Bum Chung* in Tibetan)
- Transformative Compassionate Breathing (*Tong Len* in Tibetan)

Vipashyana[9] ("mindfulness") is more completely called *Shamatha/ Vipashyana*. *Shamatha* is an intentional calming, "calm abiding," that uses various methods to focus attention, most prevalently the breath. A focus on ordinary breathing enables the practitioner to shift attention from the relative chaos of the mind to the stability of open awareness, which doesn't move, being free of mind and its disturbances. When attention is focused on awareness, *Vipashyana* arises, "insight," "panoramic awareness," "extraordinary seeing," inherent capabilities usually obscured or blocked by the random, uncontrolled, free play of the mind. The mind is vulnerable to the anxious conditions of life, and "running on automatic pilot" can be the basis of various psychological problems and disease conditions. Applying awareness-based *Vipashyana* to the mind is a practice of calming and healing and a return to more capable and integrated mind-body function.

Vase Breathing *(Bum Chung)* is *Vipashyana* practiced on the basis of a nonordinary sense of body and breathing. It is distinctly different from *Vipashyana* with respect to what breathes and what is breathed. The same profound psychological shift from mind to

---

9. Western readers may be more familiar with the term *Vipassana*, referring to essentially the same practice.

awareness is practiced, but the shift back to inherent awareness is made on the basis of breathing energy into the energy body. This will be described in substantial detail later in this book. For now we should understand that it's been necessary to extend our sense of human anatomical design and function to see that there is an inner body, the so-called energy body, inseparable from the physical body and inherent to its function, as described in popular literature by Caroline Myss (1994), and more extensively described in the literature of various meditation science traditions. This practice is doubly transformative. It is transformative with respect to what the body and its capabilities are, and it is transformative with respect to breathing. This can be viewed as an even more profound health care practice than *Vipashyana.*

Transformative Compassionate Breathing *(Tong Len)*, like Vase Breathing, is based on an extraordinary sense of body and breathing. Using visualization and observation, the practice offers self-care, a time-honored healing method with which people can heal themselves in two ways: by entering their self-healing potential with a venerated healing method, and by experiencing the remarkable health benefits of extending compassionate care to others through the medium of the breath. This practice will be disclosed more fully later in this book.

Ancient Wisdom,
New Possibilities for Healing

THROUGH THE CENTURIES and around the world, people have discovered and practiced a variety of methods with profound healing potential. So today, with our panoramic knowledge of human history and cultures, we are able to observe and select from a treasury of proven methods and understandings of profound value to human health care. And, in the process, we may discover a new understanding of how the human body functions.

References

Chopra, Deepak. *Creating Health*. Boston: Houghton-Mifflin, 1987.

————. *Quantum Healing*. New York: Bantam, 1990.

Clifford, Terry. *Tibetan Buddhist Medicine and Psychiatry: The Diamond Healing*. York Beach, ME: Samuel Weiser, Inc, 1984.

Dudjom Rinpoche. *Counsels from My Heart*. Boston: Shambhala, 1991.

Eliade, Mircea. *Shamanism*. Princeton, NJ: Princeton University Press, 1964.

Harner, Michael. *The Way of the Shaman*. San Francisco: HarperSanFrancisco, 1991.

Holmes, Ernest. *The Science of Mind*. New York: Tarcher/Putnam, 1925, 2000.

Isherwood, Christopher, and Swami Prabhavananda. *How to Know God: The Yoga Aphorisms of Patanjali*. Los Angeles: Vedanta Press, 1953.

Miller, Ruth L. *150 Years of Healing*. Portland, OR: Abib, 2000; Beaverton, OR: WiseWoman Press, 2006.

Murphy, Michael. *The Future of the Body*. New York: Tarcher/Putnam, 1992.

Myss, Caroline, *The Anatomy of the Spirit*. New York: Harmony Books, 1994.

Parfitt, Will. *The Elements of the Qabalah*. New York: Arkana/Penguin, 1994.

Roth, Ron, and P. Occhiogroso. *Prayer and the Five Stages of Healing*. Los Angeles: Hay House, 2000.

Tsogyal, Yeshe. *The Lotus-Born: The Life Story of Padmasambhava*. Boston: Shambhala, 1993.

————. *Sky Dancer*. London: Routledge and Kegan, 1984.

Yogananda, Paramahansa. *Autobiography of a Yogi*. Los Angeles: Self-Realization Fellowship, 1946.

CHAPTER 3

Meditation Research in the United States

> While meditation can be considered as a cognitive strategy by which consciousness gains control over normally non-conscious states of awareness, including involuntary bodily processes, the physiology of meditation has received more attention than any other subject from Western scientists quite out of proportion to all other dimensions of meditative experience. (Murphy 1992, 45)

CLEARLY, THE HISTORY OF MEDITATION and its use in healing is very old, very deep in our human heritage. Its visible emergence in Western scientific cultures, however, has occurred only in the past 100 years. From the 1920s onward in India, at Lonavla near Bombay, there was a major center for meditation and medicine. Using a system of physical culture and yogic therapies for many afflictions, it had support from the governments of British India and England, the Indian Health Agency, and American foundations. This *yoga* therapy center was also a research center. Its studies began a process ensuring that America would become an important center of mind-body medicine and meditation research.

Also in India, from the 1930s into the 1950s, dramatic demonstrations of the power of meditation over vital functions were documented. In each case there was a *yogi* who wanted to demonstrate for science a higher human order of function (Murphy 1992, 33). One *yogi* was buried completely, with more than 10,000 people watching. He was covered with earth and wood for eight days, without oxygen.

Many television dramas illustrate how the ER trauma team works on people who have been oxygen-deprived for even a few minutes. It's understood that without oxygen the brain will lose function and can die quickly. After a period of forty-five minutes to an hour of dramatic measures, including electric shock and stimulants, the doctors call it "time of death . . ."

Amazingly, however, after an hour, the buried *yogis* were just beginning to get into their meditation demonstration. One came out after two days, stood, and then did *yogic* handstands. The one who was completely buried for eight days had gone from a heart rate of fifty beats per minute after twenty-nine hours of burial to a rapid drop-off to no perceptible heart beat, where it remained until one-half hour before the agreed time the *yogi* was to be removed. Apparently the *yogi* had an internal clock running during his deep black burial as well as an extraordinary control of his breath and his heart (Murphy and Donovan 1999, 39ff.).

These buried *yogis* mostly came out smiling, and the question was raised, how did the *yogi* live? What did the *yogi* do?

Meditation Practice in America

THERE HAS ALWAYS BEEN a flow into America of people devoted to various religions and spiritual practices. In 1950, D. T. Suzuki came to the U.S., settled in New York, and slowly helped establish *Zen* meditation in America. *Zen* means meditation, "psychological method." *Zen* offers a simple and direct method to shift function, a sitting method bound to have various medical applications today.

In the 1960s, two physicians at the University of Tokyo studied brain-wave changes during meditation by *Zen* teachers and their disciples from the Soto and Rinzai *Zen* centers. Pulse rates, respiration, galvanic skin response, and electrical information were given by good-natured advanced and less advanced practitioners, who clearly saw that they could help science understand meditation. In these studies, four stages of meditation were observed, each measured in terms of the brain-wave patterns that showed up on electroencephalograms (EEGs).

Stage 1: Characterized by the appearance of alpha waves (the brain-wave pattern associated with dreaming, daydreaming, and being "in the zone").

Stage 2: Increase in amplitude of persistent alpha waves (associated with a stronger sense of being "in the zone").

Stage 3: Decrease in alpha-wave frequency (associated with relaxation).

Stage 4: The appearance of rhythmical theta trains (the brain-wave pattern associated with deep rest).

These findings indicate that *Zen* practice promotes a serene, alert awareness that is consistently responsive to both external and internal stimuli (Murphy and Donovan 1999, 41).

Between 1970 and 1972, at Harvard University Medical School, Herbert Benson, MD, a cardiologist with strong mind-body medicine inclinations, published several influential articles on the biology of meditation. Benson went to Asia on several occasions to study the biology of adept *Vajrayana* (Tibetan) Buddhist practitioners, and observed evidence of life-enhancement through control of vital processes (Benson 1996, 163ff.). He studied various meditation methods and was particularly impressed by the now famous *tummo*, Wisdom Fire practice. He observed several Buddhist *yogis* go out into a subzero Himalayan night wearing nothing but a cotton cloth. After sitting and developing the *tummo* heat, they were covered with wet sheets. They showed their Wisdom Fire capability by drying as many as several sheets in one night. As a result of this and other experiences, Benson saw that meditation offered remarkable biological benefits and went on to study various meditation methods, ready to qualify and quantify these benefits for medical science.

In 1975, Dr. Benson published a well-received nontechnical book, *The Relaxation Response.* It used simple, meaningful language that gave people a method with significant health benefits. For his Western audience, he replaced the word *meditation* with a new term, describing the shift of function to a hypometabolic, or internally slowed, state that was experienced in his laboratory, and called this state the Relaxation Response (RR). He pointed out that practicing the characteristics of the RR state (for example, slow, deep breathing) can elicit the state, and he encouraged people to do this practice as part of a healing process he called "wellness remembered." This was a new kind of medicine, potentially more valuable to health care than even he could imagine.

Characteristics of the Relaxation Response

AT HARVARD'S MIND/BODY CLINIC, established by Benson in September 1981, with Dr. Joan Borysenko as director, Dr. Benson has given us both research and a method. The practice is as follows:

Step 1: Pick a focus word or short phrase that's firmly rooted in your belief system.

Step 2: Sit quietly in a comfortable position.

Step 3: Close your eyes.

Step 4: Relax your muscles.

Step 5: Breathe slowly and naturally, and as you do, repeat your focus word, phrase, or prayer silently to yourself as you exhale.

Step 6: Assume a passive attitude. Don't worry about how well you're doing. When other thoughts come to mind, simply say to yourself, "Oh well," and gently return to the repetition.

Step 7: Continue for ten to twenty minutes.

Step 8: Do not stand immediately. Continue sitting quietly for a minute or so, allowing other thoughts to return. Then open your eyes and sit for another minute before rising.

Step 9: Practice this technique once or twice daily.

Benson proved that the practice of this simple but sound method improves biologic function. Meditation lowers blood pressure, slows heart rate, and reduces oxygen consumption. It rests metabolic activity, leaving more oxygen available for other functions. "As far as science knows, the calming effects of the relaxation response cannot be brought about as dramatically or as quickly by any other means" (Benson 1996, 132).

Borysenko observed some of the characteristics of those engaged in this meditation practice as follows:

> Breathing rate and oxygen consumption decline because of the profound decrease in the need for energy. Brain waves shift from an alert beta-rhythm to a relaxed alpha-rhythm ... Blood flow to the muscles decreases, and instead, blood is sent to the brain and skin, producing a feeling of warmth and rested mental alertness. It was by learning to induce the relaxation response that I began to reverse symptoms that were severe enough to send me to the emergency room. (Borysenko 1988, 13)

Meditation Is Established in American Culture

QUIETLY, AS DR. BENSON WAS WORKING, the presence of Buddhist meditation masters in the West was increasing. Like light entering a dark chemical process and changing it, irreversibly, the light of inner stillness entered the still-dark era of Cold War Western society, through the 1970s and 1980s, during the advent of AIDS and amid the still-unreleased stress of persistent thermonuclear threat.

It began with the advent of *Zen* Buddhism in New York City referred to above. By 1970, D. T. Suzuki Roshi and Chögyam Trungpa Rinpoche were teaching meditation in several American cities, and Maharishi Mahesh Yogi's Hindu-based Transcendental Meditation (TM) was being taught across the country. Since then there has been a progressive increase in the number of meditation centers in America, of every denomination.

Through the 1970s both Chögyam Trungpa Rinpoche,[10] founder of Naropa Institute, and Dudjom Rinpoche, head of the *Nyingma* lineage of Tibetan Buddhism and a meditation teacher to the Dalai Lama, were living and teaching in America. So, through the 1970s two very similar psychological methods, Japanese *Zen* and Tibetan *Vipashyana* (mindfulness-insight) meditation, found increasing respect in America. The authenticity of their methods was unmistakable. Buddhism is a science of human development, and both the lay public and medical professionals were finding that Buddhist meditation methods worked, in America, as a natural, healthy response to many basic health challenges.

Among the various forms of meditation in use in the West since that time, two forms have been widely used and researched: mindfulness meditation methods such as *Vipashyana*, and Transcendental Meditation (TM). Mindfulness meditation is a silent psychological method in which attention is shifted from mind to awareness, which becomes a therapeutic process, slowing breathing down, providing significant psychological and biological benefits. TM is a mantra-based technique, in which the practitioner focuses attention on the

---

10. The term *Rinpoche* is Tibetan for "cherished, precious" and is used as a title for a beloved teacher.

repetition of a Sanskrit word or phrase, making the practice more internally active than mindfulness meditation, but also shifting attention away from the disorder of the mind into a new state of consciousness, free of ordinary limitations, calming physiological processes.

Clinical Research

BOSTON AREA HOSPITALS have a heritage of being in the fore-front of medical advances, and the Buddhist teachers were interested in Western medicine. In 1979, Jon Kabat-Zinn established the Mindfulness-Based Stress Reduction (MBSR) clinic at the University of Massachusetts Medical Center (UMMC), the Boston area's fourth largest hospital. In 1981, Herbert Benson established the Mind/Body Clinic of the Harvard Medical School at Boston Deaconess Hospital.

The two programs continue today as outstanding clinical and research programs exploring the medical uses of meditation. The UMMC clinical program influenced the Harvard program and has been the model for hundreds of clinical programs in meditation in hospitals and medical centers throughout the United States and Canada. This kind of medicine doesn't have a lobby but it does have large public support and is the most proven of the "alternative" medicines. Of the thousands of people who have participated in the UMMC and Harvard Medical Center programs (more than 20,000 between the two of them), most have been under medical insurance coverage, which indicates some level of institutional support for this practical and clinically proven medical method. Also, many health care providers have attended the meditation-medicine programs, both to learn methods that could help their patients and for the sake of their own well-being.

The UMMC Research

The success of the UMMC program is very impressive. From 1979 to this writing, more than 18,000 people are graduates of the program, most of them under medical insurance coverage, and most of them experiencing remarkable reductions in symptoms of a wide range of diseases, including cancer, AIDS, heart disease, diabetes, and anxiety disorder.

Jon Kabat-Zinn, the developer and director of the UMMC program, has told the story of its development and given us a summary of its research observations in *Full Catastrophe Living*. He describes a sitting meditation method, Mindfulness-Insight meditation, that clearly has the ability to bring its practitioners "to a new order of reality" (Pelletier 1975, 226), bringing them in touch with the universe and the great potential of human evolution. The UMMC program offers people methods to shift to a new level of functioning and raise the quality of both health and life.

The method of meditation in the UMMC model uses breathing as a key to pain management and symptom reduction. The practice that is the cornerstone of the UMMC program may be outlined as follows:

Step 1: Sit quietly in a comfortable position.

Step 2: Eyes may be open or closed.

Step 3: Relax your muscles.

Step 4: Let your attention follow your breath, being particularly attentive to the relaxing out-breath and the moment of gap or stillness before the next breath.

Step 5: Breathe slowly and naturally. Belly breathing is best: breathe down and calm down.

Step 6: Recognize your thoughts, the anxious movement of the mind. Return to open awareness. Return to calm.

Steps 7–9: Same as the Relaxation Response.

With this and related methods, Kabat-Zinn observes symptom reduction and health development in a variety of major disease conditions, with patients reporting significant benefits in treating cancer, pain, and anxiety.

One major observation of the UMMC research is that meditation stimulates the pineal gland, located on the brain between the eyes, to produce elevated levels of melatonin, a most important hormone that is necessary to experiencing optimal function, optimal health. Among other things, melatonin is a powerful antioxidant, enhancing immune function.

Kabat-Zinn is very effective in his presentation of mindfulness as a medical method. His program inspires people to meditate and to help themselves with their health problems. People participating in the UMMC program learn to calm their body and mind to find inner balance in the face of the challenging disturbances of life. The obvious benefits help people commit to keep meditation at the heart of their life.

The UMMC uses the classical mindfulness of breath as the basis of shifting from mind to awareness. Working with breathing is a key to all the UMMC program methods: sitting and reclining meditation, *yoga*, and walking meditation. The breath is very helpful for focusing attention. Belly breathing is good for maintaining calm and awareness.

> The mind will challenge you to keep you from calm breathing, but people find that they can stay with deep breathing and calm down. If we follow the breath as a path, it has the power to help us balance body and mind. (Kabat-Zinn 1990, 61)

The Harvard Research

In 1981, when the Harvard Mind/Body Clinic was established, Benson concluded, having spent years studying the medical uses of meditation, that he had amassed "significant evidence of the tremendous diversity of medical conditions that the elicitation [Relaxation Response] together with other self-care strategies ... can heal or cure" (Benson 1996, 146).

Specific gains that he identified from the use of meditation can be considered in three categories:

- self-awareness and attention
- distinct physiological shifts
- energetic enhancement

Most long-term meditators or practitioners of the Relaxation Response have experienced benefits in one or all of these areas.

Some of the more important medical benefits of meditation observed in Benson's Mind/Body Clinic research include:

- Patients with hypertension experienced significant decreases in blood pressure and needed fewer or no medications over a three-year measurement period.

- Patients with chronic pain experienced less severity of pain, more activity, less anxiety, less depression, and less anger, and they visited the managed care facility where they received care 36 percent less often in the two years after completing the program than they did prior to treatment.

- Patients with cancer and AIDS experienced decreased symptoms and better control of nausea and vomiting associated with chemotherapy.

- Patients who suffered from anxiety or mild or moderate depression were less anxious, depressed, angry, and hostile.

- Patients undergoing painful X-ray procedures experienced less anxiety and pain and needed one-third the amount of pain and anxiety medications usually required.

- Working people experienced reduced symptoms of depression, anxiety, and hostility and had remarkably fewer medical symptoms.

- Patients who had open-heart surgery had fewer postoperative cardiac arrhythmias and less anxiety following surgery.

Transcendental Meditation Research

Perhaps the most numerous studies of meditation and its benefits are those focusing on a simple meditation practice introduced in the United States in the late 1960s by the Hindu teacher, Maharishi Mahesh Yogi, called Transcendental Meditation (TM). More than 500 published articles, involving thousands of meditators, are abstracted on the TM website (www.tm.org), alone.

The first research on the Transcendental Meditation technique, conducted at UCLA and Harvard medical schools, was published from 1970 to 1972 in the respected journals *Science, American Journal of Physiology,* and *Scientific American.* These landmark studies revealed that the Transcendental Meditation technique produced a unique state of mind and body called "restful alertness."

> ... the mind settles down to its most silent level. Since the mind and body are intimately connected, as the mind settles down the body also settles down to a deep state of rest.
>
> Researchers discovered significant reductions in respiration, minute ventilation, tidal volume, and blood lactate, and significant increases in basal skin resistance. All of these physiological measures represent a state of deep relaxation, even deeper than sleep. And they found that even though the body is in a state of deep rest, the mind is alert rather than asleep, indicated by an increased abundance of alpha waves in the EEG.... For the past 30 years, many other researchers have confirmed and expanded upon this initial research ... the experience ... is correlated with greater creativity, improved learning, higher IQ, better grades, higher moral reasoning, increased brainwave coherence, and improved neurological functioning of the body. (www.tm.org)

The practice is simple. All TM students are given a unique *mantra*—a Sanskrit word or phrase—that is intended to assist them in releasing their particular pattern of thought and feeling. They are guided through a process of relaxing the body and repeating the mantra, then sent home to perform the practice for twenty minutes, morning and evening. The initial training is sufficient for most, but it is possible to take advanced trainings, ultimately learning to train others. Through these trainings, students are encouraged to simply focus on repeating the mantra, silently, and to return to the mantra whenever they notice other thoughts or images. "Like bubbles of air in the ocean, simply watch any thoughts that bubble up as they go by, without letting them affect you," said Maharishi in one of his question-and-answer sessions.

Based on ongoing studies, the TM organization publishes the following list of benefits for people doing the practice:

- It's Easy and Enjoyable: People of all ages, cultures, and educational backgrounds can practice this simple, natural, effortless technique while sitting comfortably for 20 minutes twice a day.

- Clearer Thinking: Develop your full mental potential, improve your memory, enhance creativity, and sharpen your intellect.

- Better Health: Become more rested and relaxed, increase immunity to disease, reverse the effects of aging, and enjoy greater energy and vitality.

- More Fulfilling Relationships: Enjoy closer friendships, increased calmness, more self-confidence, and less anxiety and stress.

- A Peaceful World: Contribute your share to world peace by reducing your own stress level and radiating an influence of harmony to your surroundings.

- Personal Growth: Experience transcendental consciousness at the quietest level of your mind, and grow toward higher states of consciousness—enlightenment. (www.tm.org)

The theory developed by TM researchers to explain these benefits is that, by focusing on repeating a properly selected mantra instead of one's normal thoughts, the mind becomes still and the brain-body system becomes more coherent in its functioning. In addition, the stilled mind begins to operate at a new level of consciousness, which they call "transcendental consciousness," that permits the meditator access to more stored memories and learned or observed skills than would otherwise be available.

Many of the published studies focus on the technique's clinical effects. Dr. Dean Ornish calls TM

> an ancient stress-management technique [that] may decrease blood vessel blockage and help people avoid a heart attack or stroke. A study published in the March 2000 issue of the journal *Stroke* shows that TM decreased the thickness of blood vessel walls, a known risk factor for stroke and heart disease.... The researchers found that two 20-minute sessions of daily TM led to a widening of the space inside the practitioners' arteries. In the comparison group, which did leisure activities instead of TM, arterial thickening continued to worsen. (www.ornish.com)

Today, more than ten million people around the world have completed the initial training, with several thousand of them going on to advanced levels. As the numbers increase, more research has been done on what is called "the Maharishi Effect," or the impact that a group of people meditating regularly has on the larger community. One study, described in the film *What the BLEEP Do We Know!?* and done in Washington, D.C., had 4,000 people meditating on a regular basis through the summer, during which period the rate of violent crime was reduced by one-third. Another study, posted on the TM website "Time series impact assessment analysis of reduced international conflict and terrorism: Effects of large assemblies of participants in the Transcendental Meditation and TM-Sidhi programs," presented at the American Political Science

Association Annual Meeting, Atlanta, Georgia, August 1989), shows a marked decrease in global terrorist activity whenever a TM conference has been held. The Maharishi University has been established to provide an opportunity for students to engage in further research into the technique and its effects and relate it to other philosophies and practices.

The Ornish Program

Dr. Dean Ornish, a cardiologist, wished to enhance the ongoing well-being of his heart patients. Seeing the effectiveness of methods like RR and TM, he developed a medical meditation program (Ornish 1990) using absorptive deep breathing, a breathing of energy, *prana*, from the universal field. "In this system we inhale not only oxygen but also energy, or *prana*. In Sanskrit, *prana* means both breath and spirit. In Latin it is *spiritus*" (ibid., 165).

Dr. Ornish's program differs from the UMMC programs in the concern with *deep* breathing. He taught people to breathe deeply, to inhale vital energy in the air and take it into their bodies.

Dr. Ornish comments on meditation:

Meditation is the practice and process of paying attention and focusing your awareness....

when you ... concentrate any form of energy, including mental energy, you gain power. When you focus your mind, you concentrate better. When you concentrate better, you perform better—you can accomplish more ...

... as you experience a profound state of relaxation, deeper even than sleep ... blood pressure decreases, your heart rate slows, your arteries dilate, you think more clearly.

... you enjoy your senses more fully ... Anything that you enjoy—food, sex, music, art, massage, and so on—is greatly enhanced by meditation.

... your mind quiets down and you experience an inner sense of peace, joy, and well-being.... Before, I thought peace of mind came from getting and doing; now, I understand that it comes from being. It is our true nature to be peaceful until we disturb it.

Finally, you may directly experience and become more aware of the transcendent interconnectedness that already exists.... Most spiritual and religious traditions are based on people who experienced God directly: Abraham, Moses, Jesus, Mohammed, and Buddha, to name only a few.... Like peace, joy, and well-being, God is not something we attain from "out there" somewhere; we realize that God is in us as us. (www.ornish.com)

Through Dr. Ornish's holistic approach, including dietary changes, exercise, and guided meditation, many people with "terminal" cases of heart disease have seen significant results and much longer life spans than would be expected under more typical medical protocols. This success has led to an overall shift in the medical profession's treatment of heart conditions.

Mindfulness Meditation

Mindfulness meditation is the basis of various Buddhist traditions, including *Vipashyana* (also known as *Vipassana*), *Zen,* and the *Shamatha/Vipashyana* practice of Tibetan *Vajrayana* Buddhism. Mindfulness meditation presented at UMMC is the "insight" meditation prevalent across India and Southeast Asia and based on 2,400 years of Buddhist tradition. There is great knowledge and experience underlying the method. Buddhism does not consider itself a religion but, rather, a science of human development. Mindfulness meditation is a psychological method based on an essential recognition of the difference between *mind* and *awareness*. This distinction is practical, definite, and transformative. It is readily understood by an increasing number of people as a useful, even essential, method for personal development and health.

Though UMMC has successfully applied mindfulness to reclining PR as one of the integral methods of its program, mindfulness meditation is primarily a sitting meditation in which the natural flow of the breath, uncontrived breathing, is used to focus attention. Practitioners are able to recognize that their attention is usually lost in the uncontrolled activity of the *mind* and that they are readily able to shift their attention out of the chaos of the mind into stable open *awareness*, distinctly free of the *mind*.

Mindfulness is a process of seeing and appreciating how things work. One psychodynamic mechanism by which mindfulness seems to work is by helping the patient to distinguish primary sensory experience (for example, chronic pain, physical symptoms of anxiety) from the secondary emotional or cognitive processes created in reaction to the primary experience. It is hypothesized that, when unrecognized, these secondary processes contribute greatly to a patient's distress (Barrows and Jacobs 2001, 10). However, in the state of enhanced awareness, one is able to distinguish between the sensation itself and the suffering that the mind creates in response to the sensation. Thus, mindfulness of pain allows one to separate the sensation from the suffering, which in turn tends to reduce anxiety and any tensions that might otherwise contribute to the pain.

Mindfulness is a calming process of concentration and flexibility of attention, simultaneously. It neither suppresses nor acts out emotions. It is a free middle path. Even though it is considered an ideal antidote to anxiety and stress, it is a new way of being rather than an antidote to mind and emotion. For awareness-based meditation, anxiety, impatience, and boredom are all good states to work with.

"Becoming aware is a human act that is so basic that it is independent of the contexts in which one becomes aware of one's own conscious activity" (Depraz, Varela, and Vermersch 2000, 1). Awareness, in most sacred traditions, is known to be primordially free of mind. It is the basis of human freedom and realization, free in the very contexts of suffering and sickness mind may find itself lost in. Mindfulness meditation is a psychological method, readily accessible to most people, that offers a direct path to aware recognition of the time-based conditions of one's life, recognition that faces time and condition but is timeless and free of condition. Present-moment awareness, free of mind's anxieties about past and future, is the basis of calming and insight *(Shamatha/Vipashyana)*.

The more that people practice the shift from anxious mind (bound by time) to awareness (timeless and open), the more they slow down time. The more they calm down, the more they slow down. The more people shift from the experience of time to the experience of timelessness, the more people tend to come to an experience of "time-stop," where they may experience breakthrough, free of time, perhaps the basis of all healing. In the non-doing of mindfulness meditation, the intentional giving up of involvement in time, people feel the boundless energy of the timeless and deathless state, unconditioned immortal awareness, ever-present. Millions of people are willingly giving up hope and fear to live free of time in the eternal presence of unobstructed life, the heart of mindfulness meditation in its different forms.

The Sitting Practice of Mindfulness

Mindfulness meditation methods are simple and elegant. First there is attention to posture. Though there are profound reclining meditations (for example, the UMMC Progressive Relaxation body scan), sitting meditation, *dhyana asana*, is the perennial and prevalent mode of meditation. If sitting on cushions or pillows or a meditation bench isn't possible, sitting in a chair is very good, especially if the participant can sit free of the back of the chair, with the spine self-supporting. If one can sit with the spine as upright as possible, effortlessly, the spine will lift a little in a natural vertical alignment.

Meditation posture can be the position of revolution. It can be a way of balancing the body "to stop the world." It can be an effortless way of sitting into potential, a way of directly sitting into life itself. Many people initially have trouble sitting in a relaxed cross-legged posture, but most people can become at ease with some kind of sitting meditation. If you sit on the floor, it's best to use a cushion to lift your sacrum higher than your knees. That will bring your body naturally into stable balance. This new balance will slow down and may stop unconscious tendencies of mind and body that support illness.

To access self-reliance and deep potential, it helps to adopt an effortless erect posture, a kind of noble posture, with head, neck, and back aligned vertically. Such posture aligns a natural vertical flow of life force. If the spine is balanced, self-supporting, and if the head is balanced over that, the spine will tend to lift a little, releasing pressure on its vertebrae and nerves, which is conducive to healing and freedom.

Sitting meditation lets you move into stillpoint, which encourages the mind to break from its relentless activity. Sitting into stillpoint facilitates the natural shift from mind to awareness, a transformative shift, a revolutionary shift. Because this posture is good for slowing down the mind, even stopping the mind, it has enabled people for centuries to access the healing return to awareness, to come back to the unlimited, all-knowing human potential.

Once seated, the breathing is the immediate concern. Awareness is placed on the breath. Thinking takes you out of the present moment, preventing you from being present, then awareness brings you back to your breath. Breath is body; body is present. The meditator keeps coming back to the breath to calm down the mind. Coming back to awareness and breath works against the reactiveness and momentum of the mind. With the method of awareness meditation one makes a "conscious effort to move in a direction of healing and inner peace. This means learning to work with the very stress and pain that is causing you to suffer" (Kabat-Zinn 1990, 2).

"We speak of the 'practice' of meditation, and the 'practice' of mindfulness, meaning the actual engagement in the discipline, the inward gesture that invites and embodies it" (Depraz, Varela, and Vermersch 2000, 15). People use the practice of mindfulness meditation to directly engage awareness in the present moment. Meditation practice has various forms, used for various periods of time, but its aim is to develop a continuity of awareness. The practice is a direct and proven path to unlimited inner resources and the source of awareness (ibid., 56–61).

Psychological Benefits of Meditation

SUMMARIZING THE RESEARCH referred to in the above sections, Murphy and Donovan (1999, 81ff.) describe the following psychological benefits of meditation:

- perceptual ability
- reaction time and physical motor skill
- field independence
- concentration and intelligence
- empathy
- creativity
- self-actualization

They observe that various meditation schools offer methods to cultivate clarity, flexibility, efficiency, and a broadened range of psychological functions. This is seen in the meditation results reviewed in the fifty-one pages of research abstracts in their book *The Physical and Psychological Effects of Meditation* (1999). Though all the above-indicated psychological benefits are important in maintaining a healthy human, with respect to pathological conditions the pain-management potential of meditation makes it an invaluable resource for many areas of medicine.

Meditation and Pain Management

Extensive research conducted at UMMC (Kabat-Zinn 1990, 77–78) demonstrated that meditation produced significant reductions in the following: present moment pain, negative body image, inhibition of activity (movement limitation), psychological disturbance, anxiety and depression, and the need for pain-related drugs. The benefits are considerably more than increased tolerance of pain.

With the mindfulness meditation method used at UMMC, people learn to distinguish between mind and awareness. As people learn to expose mind to awareness, they learn to see how the mind dwells on anxiety and fear and burns up energy, exhausting them, limiting their ability and reserves. With mindfulness meditation they learn that they're capable of staying in the present moment, even while experiencing high levels of pain. They see that their mind likes to avoid being present by making a big deal about the pain and creating the experience of suffering. They see that for healthy reasons they want to stay in open awareness and avoid mind's creation of suffering.

People practicing mindfulness meditation see that they can develop fearlessness and gain energy by distinguishing between pain sensations and what the mind is trying to do with them. They avoid letting their mind agonize and waste energy reserves. They see that they have a choice to prevent distress and build courage and inner strength in the process. They learn that staying with present-moment pain naturally releases endorphins, the body's natural painkillers, which then increase the ability to stay present.

The more one is present with the sensation, the higher the endorphin levels and the greater the development of fearlessness. This heals those situations in which suffering weakens reserves and encourages an attitude that fosters health. With psychiatric and pain management drugs costing more than a hundred billion dollars a year, we have many reasons to ask medical science to advance the use of the medical art of meditation.

Physiological Benefits of Meditation

EXTENSIVE RESEARCH HAS SHOWN that significant biological and psychological problems are directly caused by anxiety and stress. In brief, anxiety causes an overproduction of the hormones adrenaline and cortisol, which suppress important biological functions in order to shift energy into muscle systems for a "fight or flight" reaction, based on old instinctive tendencies, no longer appropriate. Anxiety suppresses immune system function primarily through elevated levels of cortisol in the bloodstream. Anxiety and stress, with accompanying hormonal imbalance, have been proved, through extensive research, to be primary factors in the weakening of health and the cause of various immune-deficiency diseases. The widespread chemical treatment of anxiety has resulted in additional biological and psychological problems.

Self-calming meditation has been shown to directly reduce adrenaline and cortisol secretion, naturally restoring hormonal balance in general and normalizing immune system function. In addition meditation produces elevated levels of the major hormones melatonin, DHEA, and serotonin, and endorphins, powerful pain-relieving, pleasure-causing agents secreted by the nervous system. Benson speaks of the direct health and medical impact of meditation as follows:

> When you focus for a short time, gently brushing aside any intrusive thoughts, your mind and body suddenly become a five star resort in which all the service personnel make your restoration and health their priority and are especially concerned with alleviating the harmful effects of stress. This great team of stress-busters and body-relaxers emerge when everyday thoughts and worries are put aside. (Benson 1996, 130)

Benefits with respect to treatment of major disease conditions, including cardiovascular disease, cancer, and others, are described elsewhere in this book. Presently our focus will be primarily on three areas: hormonal balance, immune system enhancement, and management of pain and anxiety. These subjects are of fundamental concern to all biopsychic disorders.

Melatonin

The fact that meditation produces elevated levels of melatonin, the hormone secreted by the pineal gland located at the center of the brain, was first disclosed by research conducted at UMMC (Kabat-Zinn 1990). The pineal gland has drawn the attention of human insight for a long time. In the seventeenth century, René Descartes, in his famous *Treatise of Man*, called the pineal gland the seat of the human psyche, the principal location of self-awareness. In sacred literature more than 3,500 years old, the *Vedas* of India described the pineal gland in the context of the energy body:

> The [pineal] gland was portrayed as one of the seven *chakras*, or centers of vital energy, which are arranged along the central axis of the body. The pineal gland was thought to be the supreme or crown chakra ... the ultimate center of spiritual force. (Reiter and Robinson 1995, 131)

While these insights are inspiring concerns for people interested in meditation, the current worldwide interest in melatonin, evident in the presence of hundreds of research papers and books on the subject, is focused on its biological benefits, particularly concerning its remarkable effects on the human immune system. Melatonin many be the most potent and versatile antioxidant. It directly stimulates interleukin-2 activity that in turn stimulates the increase of all the various cells of the immune system, in a pervasive optimization of immune function, and directly restores and increases T-helper cell production in bone marrow. As a result, it has been used as a therapeutic agent in cancer and AIDS therapy.

Melatonin is known to have a calming effect, bringing contentment and improved mood. In stress-inducing times, which tend to cause detrimental imbalances, melatonin is renowned as a sleep aid. Especially when produced naturally to elevated levels, it makes normal sleep and rest possible even in challenging situations. Together with DHEA, serotonin, and endorphins, a raised level of melatonin is an important reason why meditation brings healthy calming balance.

DHEA (dehydroepiandrosterone)

DHEA, produced in the adrenal glands, just above the kidneys, is the most plentiful human hormone and is essential for health. Like melatonin, it tends to diminish in the body as people age. An increased level of life-enhancing DHEA in older meditation practitioners was one of the first biological benefits of meditation to be observed.

Like melatonin, DHEA has a variety of health-increasing benefits. It is an immunity enhancement agent that has been proved to be beneficial in the prevention and treatment of cancer, cardiovascular disease, diabetes, lupus, and other disorders. DHEA stimulates the production of monocytes (T-cells and B-cells), potent immunity biochemicals that cause the production of other immune system agents. T-cells (white blood cells produced in the bone marrow) produce two powerful immune system agents—interleukin-2 and gamma interferon—intelligent defense agents that help maintain health.

DHEA is good for the bones, muscles, blood pressure, vision, and hearing. It is the substance from which the male and female hormones are developed. It's probably the essential reason that kidney *chi* is an important concern in Chinese medicine. DHEA contributes to vitality and youthfulness. It's a mood elevator that makes people feel and look better. It enhances brain biochemistry and growth. Anxiety and stress lower normal DHEA levels in the bloodstream, while meditation elevates DHEA levels.

Endorphins

Meditation is also known to increase levels of endorphins, a set of peptides secreted throughout the nervous system that have very strong pain-relieving and pleasure-inducing effects, similar to morphine. Of these powerful chemicals, endocrinologist Deepak Chopra writes:

> Thus the brain [and nervous system in general] produces narcotics up to 200 times stronger than anything you can buy ... with the added boon that our own pain-killers are non-addictive. Morphine and endorphins both block pain by filling a certain receptor on the neuron and preventing other chemicals that carry the message of pain from coming in, without which there can be no sensation of pain, no matter how much physical provocation is present. (Chopra 1990, 62)

The above four vital biological substances contribute to immune system strength and personal feelings of well-being, essential for disease prevention, recovery, and maintaining health.

Meditation as a Means for Promoting Well-Being

The words medicine and meditation come from the same root, the Latin word *mediere,* meaning "to cure," and meditation has always had a close alignment with healing. *Medi*cine = curing the results of a condition; *Medit*ation = taking out the basis of any condition. Medicine cures by eliminating the symptoms of a disorder. Meditation goes deeper, restoring homeostasis through "right inward measure," which is one definition of healing.

Kenneth Pelletier, MD, published his excellent book on mind-body medicine, *Mind as Healer/Mind as Slayer*, in 1975. In Part Four he describes meditation as "psychologically and physiologically more refreshing and energy restoring than sleep" (197). He defines two basic methods of meditation, through which the practitioner may come to a psychological state called *satori*, or transcendental awareness: (1) focusing of attention on an object of meditation, such as a mantra or a psychological process, such as breathing; and (2) opening up of attention, such as in *Zen* or *Vipashyana* meditation, which use focus on the flow of the breath as a basis for staying open (Pelletier 1975, 192).

The object of both kinds of meditation methods, Pelletier says (193), is to gain mastery over attention. That is the key to a shift of function and direction in health. Awareness of mind, awareness of thought, awareness of anxiety is key to the quality of the Benson technique as it is of meditation in general. So, though TM has produced a large and significant body of research in support of the health-supporting effects of its mantra-based methods, it's the research concerned with *Zen* (Direct Awareness) and *Vipashyana* (Insight) meditation that provides the basis for the advanced medical applications and methods we shall offer in this book.

The healing qualities of meditation documented across all the research include:

- Intervention: Meditation is well documented as an intervention reducing the effects of many conditions.

- Empowerment: Discipline empowers; commitment to an ongoing practice is essential; it enables people to develop inner resources, to be progressively less limited by conditioning, to touch upon the resources potential in the unconditioned state.

- Symptom Reduction: Meditation brings significant reductions in many medical and psychological symptoms; but in addition, people change for the better, which is healing, beyond body and mind.

- Enduring Effects: In the UMMC program the changes produced over eight weeks lasted up to three years without continuity of the practices. However, 85 percent of the participants continue the practices.

- Behavioral Shifts: Meditation encourages conscious action. It keeps people out of emergency rooms and off mind-dulling addictive chemical agents as they take on new, consciously chosen behaviors.

Because of these qualities, meditation has been found to be useful in the treatment of a variety of chronic conditions, including asthma (Goleman 1995, 76), fibromyalgia (ibid.), insomnia (Benson 1996, 146), migraine and cluster headaches (ibid.), and infertility (ibid.). The above characteristics of meditation are useful in what are usually considered terminal situations, as well.

The American Medical Association website (www.ama-assn.org) lists the major causes of death as follows:

- cardiovascular and heart disease (including stroke)

- cancer

- hospital care (in the form of adverse drug reactions and death from surgery)

Meditation practices have been proved to ease each of the above conditions, as we shall explore in the following sections.

Cardiovascular Concerns

Cardiovascular disease, especially stroke, is the greatest health concern in America and in the West in general. The dietary causes are well documented (Ornish 1990). Concerning the psychological and emotional causes of cardiovascular problems, we know this: We don't usually respond to stressful situations physically, and because people don't burn up the energy released by the fight-or-flight reaction, they are vulnerable to various negative consequences

(Benson 1996, 128). Meditation is an antidote for cardiovascular problems as follows:

Stress and anxiety call for greater blood flow, more forceful heart beats, and higher blood pressure. Meditation moderates heart beat and lowers blood pressure.

Higher blood pressure strains and enlarges the heart. It also contributes to the blockage of the arteries, arteriosclerosis. The high blood pressure and blockages lead to the bursting of arteries, causing stroke and internal bleeding. Regular meditation can prevent and reverse heart disease (Ornish, 1990).

Adrenaline caused by anxiety and stress can disturb the heart rhythms, causing cardiac arrhythmias. Meditation balances heart beat irregularities.

Anxiety and stress lower people's threshold of pain, which may cause other problems. Meditation increases tolerance of pain.

Cardiovascular problems then cause greater anxiety, depression, and anger. Long-term stress and anxiety can be a vicious circle for the heart. Meditation breaks habitual patterns, releasing emotional factors.

In *Emotional Intelligence* (1995), Daniel Goleman describes the following dangers of chronic anger:

- faster heart rate and higher blood pressure over the years
- resulting in a buildup of plaque in the arteries, causing coronary heart disease and blood clotting
- leading to myocardial infarction (heart attack) and stroke

In this age of high anxiety and stress, "... chronic hostility and repeated episodes of anger seem to put men at greatest risk for heart disease" (ibid., 173).

Goleman suggests that depression may be another major emotional cause of heart disease: "Noting that depression increases fivefold the likelihood of coronary heart disease, that kind of patient is at high risk. It's unethical to not start trying to treat these factors" (ibid., 185). Meditation is a known treatment for depression (Benson 1996, 147).

The evidence for meditation as an indicated intervention in both the prevention and treatment of heart disease is well established. Meditation is a widely known reducer of anxiety and stress. Benson said that people who meditate recover from stressful impacts faster, and they have fewer chronic or inappropriate emergency responses (ibid., 57). Calm presence of mind in people who practice meditation brings appropriate behavior.

Pelletier has observed that meditation is effective because it inhibits the negative patterns established within the sympathetic nervous system.

> Meditation breaks the patterns of incessant sympathetic arousal that are a correlate of anxiety states and is implicated in a range of stress related disorders ranging from hypertension to cancer. (Pelletier 1975, 192)

In the survey of the research literature on the effects of meditation cited in Murphy and Donovan's book (1999), we find substantial evidence that meditation lowers heart rate, lowers blood pressure in people who are normal to moderately hypertensive, and normalizes irregularities of heart rhythm (45–57). With respect to blood flow, they conclude:

> Meditation often helps relax the large muscle groups pressing on the circulatory system in various parts of the body. It might also relax the small muscles that control the vessels themselves; when that happens, the resulting elasticity of blood vessel walls would help reduce the pressure inside them. (ibid., 50)

The heart rates of both experienced and inexperienced meditators recovered from stressor impacts more quickly than control subjects, demonstrating a psychophysical configuration in stress situations opposite to that seen in stress-related syndromes ... Meditation generally produces psychological results opposite from those of stress. (Goleman and Schwartz 1976, 456)

From the above it is evident that meditation is a proven method of cardiovascular disease prevention and treatment. Though some cardiovascular treatment plans indicate meditation as a significant therapeutic component, given the expense and limitation of the value of surgical and chemical treatment of heart disease, and given the minimal expense and great potential of meditation as a heart disease prevention and therapy, a shift to a more effective medical paradigm clearly would include significant increases in application of meditation in heart care and a corresponding increase in research into its benefits in cardiovascular care.

Cancer

Though the causes of cancer may be less clear than the causes of heart disease, there is some evidence that anxiety and fear, particularly in women, may be significant factors, as they are well known to impair immune function.

The extensive research at UMMC cited in this chapter has clearly established meditation as a proven method of anxiety and stress reduction and enhancement of melatonin production, and the benefits associated with the reduction of cardiovascular concerns described in the preceding section are applicable to the immune system as a whole. These results suggest that meditation can play a significant role in the treatment of cancer, in addition to any surgical, chemical, or radiation treatment employed.

> Magarey (1981b, 1983) stated that medical technology has not reduced the death rate from cancer for 50 years, suggesting that a broader, more holistic approach, involving meditation is indicated. He pointed out that meditation is associated with physiological rest and stability, and also with the reduction of psychological stress and the development of a more positive attitude toward life, with an inner sense of calm, strength and fulfillment. (Murphy and Donovan 1999, 76)

In the more than twenty years since Magarey published the above statements concerning cancer, the death rate from cancer is relatively unchanged, but there has been an increase of the use of meditation in cancer therapy and there is now a better understanding of why it is indicated in cancer care. Murphy and Donovan cite a number of studies, including the following:

Meares proposed a form of intensive meditation associated with the regression of cancer (1983); discussed the relationship between stress, meditation, and cancer (1982a, 1982b); reported on a case of regression of recurrence of carcinoma of the breast at a mastectomy site associated with intensive meditation (1981); reported the results of treatment of seventy-three patients with advanced cancer who attended at least twenty sessions of meditation and experienced significant reductions of anxiety and depression (1980a); reported on a case of remission of massive metastasis from undifferentiated carcinoma of the lung associated with intensive meditation (1980b); analyzed meditation as a psychological approach to cancer treatment (1979b); reported on a case of regression of cancer of the rectum after intensive meditation (1979a); analyzed the quality of meditation effective in the regression of cancer (1978a); reported on the regression of osteogenic sarcoma metastases associated with intensive meditation (1978c); looked at the relationship between vivid visualization and dim visual awareness in the regression of cancer after meditation (1978a); raised the issue of atavistic regression, which reportedly occurs in meditation, as a factor in the remission of cancer (1977); and reported on the case of a woman whose breast cancer was alleviated through intensive meditation (1976a). Gersten (1978) reported the case of a forty-three-year-old patient who used meditation as a treatment of last resort for diplopia and ataxia. Although the reason for the improvement his patient experienced in these diseases is elusive, Gersten believed that meditation was a significant factor in the healing process. (ibid., 77)

Most importantly, in understanding the potential of mind-body medicine, we see that our potential for control over our somatic systems is greater than had been previously understood. Like biofeedback, the meditation experience can demonstrate to patients that they are capable of producing a shift in the body's functioning—a profound change in their relationship to their body. Seeing that they have a measure of control over function can be both exhilarating and therapeutic. "Functions thought to be beyond conscious control were quite controllable with specialized practice" (Achterberg 1985, 196).

Meditation methods are biologically beneficial both because they give us a sense of control over biological process and, at the same time, because they give us detachment from the processes of mind that often impair our physiological function.

> ... reaching a detached state of mind for even 5 minutes a day is so valuable that it can infuse your body with the equivalent energy of 6 months of living in hope. [It's] a way of separating yourself from the fears of mind and viewing your circumstance as an experience through which you are passing rather than one that controls your physical life. (Myss 1997, 160)

Hospital Care

In order to reduce fatalities and extended debility from surgery and overmedication, hospitals have increasingly been introducing meditation programs for surgery patients.

> Every surgeon knows that people who are extremely scared do terribly in surgery. They bleed too much; they have more infections and complications. They have a harder time recov-

ering. It's much better if they are calm ... Panic and anxiety hike blood pressure and veins distended by blood pressure bleed more profusely when cut by the surgeon's knife. Excess bleeding is one of the most troublesome complications and can lead to death. (Dossey 1992, 164)

With respect to adverse drug reactions (ADR), it is well proved that meditation is a remarkable pain management therapy; practitioners of meditation require less or no pain medication, thereby reducing drug intake that may be an ADR factor.

Diabetes

Diabetes is another major cause of death in the West. It is an increasing health problem in developing countries, as well, where populations are shifting from traditional, vegetable and whole-grain oriented diets to the commercial Western diet, based on sugars, fats, salts, and starches. Such a diet exacts a toll on the pancreas, leading to insulin imbalances and ultimately the symptoms of diabetes. Because blood flow and oxygenation are affected by meditation, and stress-related insulin-secretions are reduced in the meditative states, positive results have been observed:

> Blood sugar levels of subjects with Type-2 diabetes practicing a meditation-relaxation technique were significantly reduced after participating in a 6-week program, whereas the blood sugar levels of subjects in a diabetes education program and a control group did not significantly change. (Goleman 1995, 76)

A Medical Approach

THE PRIMARY THESIS OF THIS BOOK is that historical events have made new therapeutic methods available, and access to knowledge of those methods is a basic right. "Knowledge can heal, and according to mind-body science, knowledge is the greatest healer of all" (Chopra 1995, 8).

The research described in this chapter indicates that meditation methods have emerged as one of those new therapies, affecting many health conditions and offering people a way to live well with the challenges of our age. Meditation methods can reduce or eliminate a variety of health disorders. Meditation is a self-applied skill, a unique medical art that can directly benefit health with no medical risk. Sitting to meditate, to relax and let the breath slow down and deepen, can be used as a complement to any allopathic medical treatment. In some cases it may be a complete medical path in itself, avoiding the risks of invasive medicine and developing the person's confidence in improving his or her own function.

Like all healing practices, it does require faith in a method to use it well. Meditation instills faith in its potential and its immediate effects. Meditation instills instinctive faith that its methods make sense and that they bring people to greater function. And most importantly, meditation restores faith in oneself, which becomes a great resource in the emerging new era of health care.

Meanwhile, faith in the Western industrial medical paradigm is clearly waning and public and scientific interest in the potential of mind-body medicine in general, and meditation in particular, has been unprecedented in our culture. In the past thirty years more than 15,000 research papers and books have been published on the use of mind-body interventions in health care. Still the corporations and institutions of reductionist "scientific" health care tenaciously hold on to their power, and, in spite of public interest in letting the alternative approaches of the new era of medicine fully emerge, they resist the birth of a new and better era. Yet the world turns and changes, seemingly even to accelerate as the new era emerges, offering more complete and profound kinds of medical care.

References

Achterberg, Jeanne. *Imagery in Healing*. Boston: Shambhala, 1985.

American Medical Association website: www.ama-assn.org.

Barrows, Kevin A., and Bradly P. Jacobs. "Mind-Body Medicine: An Introduction and Review of the Literature," draft, September 2001.

Benson, Herbert. *The Relaxation Response*. New York: William Morrow & Co., 1975.

———. *Timeless Healing: Optimal Medicine, Optimal Health*. New York: Scribner, 1996.

Borysenko, Joan. *Minding the Body, Mending the Mind*. New York: Bantam, 1988.

Chopra, Deepak. *Boundless Energy*. New York: Harmony Books, 1995.

———. *Quantum Healing*. New York: Bantam, 1990.

Depraz, Natalie, Francisco Varela, and Pierre Vermersch. *On Becoming Aware: A Pragmatics of Experiencing*. Vol. 43 in Advances in Consciousness Research. John Benjamins Publishing Company, 2000.

Dossey, Larry. *Meaning and Medicine*. New York: Bantam, 1992.

Goleman, Daniel. *Emotional Intelligence*. New York: Bantam, 1995.

Goleman, Daniel, and G. E. Schwartz. "Meditation as an Intervention in Stress Reactivity." *Journal of Consulting and Clinical Psychology* 44, no. 3 (1976): 456–66.

Jacobson, Edmund. *Progressive Relaxation*. Chicago: University of Chicago Press, 1938.

Kabat-Zinn, Jon. *Full Catastrophe Living*. New York: Bantam-Doubleday, 1990.

Magarey, C. "Anxiety, Fear, and Meditation." *Medical Journal of Australia* 1, no. 7 (1981): 375.

Murphy, Michael. *The Future of the Body*. Los Angeles: Tarcher, 1992.

Murphy, Michael, and Steven Donovan. *Physical and Psychological Effects of Meditation*. Sausalito, CA: IONS, 1999.

Myss, Caroline.*Why People Don't Heal, and How They Can.* New York: Harmony Books, 1997.

Ornish, Dean. *Program for Reversing Heart Disease.* New York: Random House, 1990.

Ornish, Dean, website: www.ornish.com.

Pelletier, Kenneth. *Mind as Healer/Mind as Slayer.* New York: Dell, 1975.

Reiter, Russel, and Jo Robinson. *Melatonin: Your Body's Natural Wonder Drug.* New York: Bantam, 1995.

Schlitz, Marilyn, et al. *Consciousness and Healing.* St. Louis, MO: Elsevier, 2005.

Suzuki, D. T. *An Introduction to Zen Buddhism.* New York: Harper & Row, 1949.

———. *Zen Buddhism.* New York: Doubleday, 1956.

Transcendental Meditation website: www.tm.org.

PART TWO

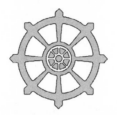

A New Model
for Healing

CHAPTER 4

States of Consciousness—
Emerging Understandings

URING THE 1960S AND EARLY 1970S, while meditation was being
introduced to America, college students and faculty were
engaged in many explorations into the effects of various chemicals
and were recording results that remarkably paralleled the descriptions shared by mystics across religious traditions down through
the centuries. As the results of all this exploration and research filtered through the psychology research community, fascinating questions were raised—questions that challenged basic assumptions
about the nature of mind and consciousness. Two opposing schools
of psychology emerged out of the process. One of these was the
structuralist-materialists, for whom all awareness, consciousness,
thought, and emotions were a product of the chemical interactions
of the brain. The other was the transpersonalists, for whom personal consciousness was the dynamic result of the interaction of
cultural, physiological, and other, not always definable, processes
going on within and around the individual.

A significant contributor to the dialogue between these groups
was a meticulous experimental psychologist at the University of
California at Davis, Dr. Charles T. Tart. He felt compelled to respond
to the phenomena going on all around him, saying:

In the last month two graduate students in physics have come to talk to me about their experiences of their "souls leaving their bodies"; a sociology graduate student told me about a group of students he meets with regularly to discuss what to do with your state of consciousness and style of life after exhausting the LSD-25 experience; a mathematics graduate student asked for a guide to the scientific literature on marijuana ... (1969, 4)

Unable to address these questions in conventional psychological terms, Tart set out to develop an experimental framework and language for identifying, describing, and predicting the processes associated with the growing body of experiential evidence.

In his early volume of readings, *Altered States of Consciousness* (1969), Tart collected some of the most precise descriptions of experiences available in the literature, exploring the nature of dream consciousness, hypnagogic states, hypnosis, and states induced by the use of psychedelic drugs. In the introduction to this collection, he states that

An altered state of consciousness [ASC] for a given individual is one in which he clearly feels a *qualitative* shift in his pattern of mental functioning, that is, he feels not just a quantitative shift (more or less alert, more or less visual imagery, ...), but also that some quality or qualities of his mental processes are *different*. (1969, 2)

According to Tart, every culture has its own attitudes toward ASCs. Some respect ASCs for potential wisdom, and some fear them. Mind has changed throughout history and attitudes toward ASCs change. In America today, the fields of psychology and psychiatry have shown insufficient interest in altered states.

In a later volume, entitled simply *States of Consciousness* (1975), Tart applies a systems approach to the material he had accumulated over nearly a decade of research to develop a model of the various states of consciousness that every individual moves through in the course of a day, or a lifetime. In the process, he comes to a new way of thinking about consciousness. He distinguishes between awareness and consciousness, saying that awareness is knowledge that something is happening, elemental perceiving or feeling. Consciousness, he says, is more complex. It's modulated by the mind. "I would use the word *awareness* to describe, for instance, my simple perception of the sound of a bird.... I would use the word *consciousness* to indicate the complex of operations that recognizes a sound as a bird call, that identifies the species of bird." (Tart 1975, 28)

As Tart continued to work with both the language and the experiences he was encountering, he developed a model that differs significantly from the familiar "conservative" understanding of mind as the product of sensory input and chemical interaction. Tart's model describes consciousness as a complex process of distinguishing and relating that is shaped by one's cultural, familial, educational, and experiential background. In his model, consciousness is informed by "pure awareness," which is "something that comes from outside the structure of the physical brain, as well as something influenced by the structure of the brain" (ibid., 29).

This idea of pure awareness as coming from outside the brain is, he says, "a most unpopular idea in scientific circles, but ... there is enough scientific evidence that consciousness is capable of temporarily existing in a way that seems independent of the physical body ..." (ibid., 30). Later, he distinguished between "awareness" and "attention," saying that the latter is "how we direct" awareness.

A second aspect of Tart's model that was "unpopular in scientific circles" is the idea that "physical reality is not a completely fixed entity, but something that may actually be shaped in some fundamental manner by the individual's beliefs about it" (ibid., 31). As an example, he refers to an experience described by Joseph Chilton Pearce in *The Crack in the Cosmic Egg* (1971) in which Pearce was temporarily convinced he was impervious to pain and "ground out

the tips of glowing cigarettes on his cheeks, palms, and eyelids ...
felt no pain, and there was no sign of physical injury" (ibid.). Tart
points out that, in material terms, the tip of a cigarette has such a
high temperature that it must burn the skin—yet the skin was not
burned; hence physical reality was shaped in some way by Pearce's
belief.

The third major contribution of Tart's model of states of consciousness is the understanding that "ordinary consciousness" is
not a particular, discrete state. What is "normal" or "ordinary"
varies from culture to culture, from individual to individual, and
from situation to situation. For example, the state of consciousness
in which we drive a car or watch television is very different from
that in which we cook a meal or repair a bicycle—they are both
waking states but use very different modes of functioning, show
very different brain-wave patterns, and light up different areas of the
brain on scanners. As a result, Tart discarded the language of
"Altered States" of consciousness and replaced it with "Discrete
States," suggesting that we experience a continuum of states of consciousness over the course of the day, each of which has its own
distinguishing characteristics. In this, Tart's work supports and
reflects that of the great pioneer of psychology, William James, who
said in a paper published in 1898,

> Our normal waking consciousness is but one special type of
> consciousness, while all about it, parted from it by the filmi-
> est of screens, there lie potential forms of consciousness
> entirely different. We may go through life without suspect-
> ing their existence, but apply the requisite stimulus and at a
> touch they are there in all their completeness. (1978, 401)

A Continuum

IF WE CONSIDER OUR EXPERIENCE over the course of a day, we can
begin to understand the various states of consciousness we move

through. Immediately prior to awaking we are usually dreaming, a state of consciousness that involves particular brain functions and has its own "laws" of operation. As we begin to awaken, we pass through a state that is called hypnagogic, in which certain areas of the sensory system function at higher levels than normal and logical; rational thought function is minimal. As we move into our day, we may sit with a beverage and become engrossed in a news story in the paper or on television—we've entered a new state of consciousness in which alpha waves dominate the brain function and the sensory system filters out unrelated external inputs. We shower, dress, and move out into the world in the "ordinary" consciousness of activity—unless we happen to have been daydreaming in the process. On the bus or train, or in the elevator, fragments and sets of thoughts shift constantly through undefined states and we are once more all but oblivious to external events, until we are startled out of our reverie—another state of consciousness—by our arrival at our destination. And so forth. Even without the use of medications, drugs, or mind-altering methods, we have already experienced several states of consciousness and we haven't even begun the day's work!

States of consciousness, then, are best understood not as "normal" and "altered," but as a continuum of mind function. Near the center of that continuum might be the states associated with conversation, completing familiar tasks, or exploring something new and interesting. At one extreme, we can place the state in which we experience pure awareness—undistracted awareness without limitation, free of the obstruction created by thought and emotion. At the other end is total distraction—that is, continual responding to every external stimulus with both emotions and evaluative processes. Daydreaming or reverie can be placed somewhere between the states in which we do our daily tasks and the experience of pure awareness. Other states, such as those associated with "the zone" in sports, or with the creative movement of dancing, would probably come between daydreaming and "pure awareness."

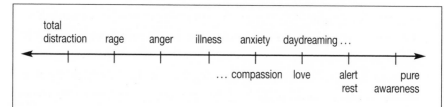

Figure 1. A continuum model of states of consciousness, from total distraction through rage, anger, illness, and anxiety, to pure awareness, by way of daydreaming, compassion, love and gratitude, and alert rest.

The states in which we experience overwhelm, anger, and upset can be placed closer to the "total distraction" extreme.

Other Western Models

I F WE LOOK AT THE HISTORY OF PSYCHOLOGY, we can see that many great thinkers have explored the nature of consciousness and mind, with some very effective models. Most of those developed in the nineteenth and twentieth centuries were attempts to explain behavioral pathologies and abnormalities. Freud's famous "ego, superego, id" model is perhaps the best known of these, but his students Carl Jung and Roberto Assagioli each came up with models that sought to explain the different forms of function and the therapeutic interventions that fit their experience. Jung's tends to be transpersonal in nature, relating the individual consciousness to a shared human, or collective, consciousness, while Assagioli's, though far more complex, tends to remain within the structural-physical realm of the individual. All of these models are useful in understanding the processes by which pathologies and other undesirable patterns develop and can be treated. None of them, however, were designed to explain the different states of consciousness that each of us experience on a moment-to-moment basis.

Another approach to consciousness was the cybernetic model of mind functioning offered by neurologist H. Ross Ashby, who used the language of cybernetics to synthesize what became the basis for a "bio-computer" model of the brain-mind system (1964). At the other extreme, Gregory Bateson took some of the same cybernetic concepts to develop "an ecology of mind," in which mental process was seen as a function of the interacting totality of the individual as part of family, workplace, culture, and ecosystem (1972).

Outside of the realm of theoretical or clinical psychology, however, another set of models has been emerging. One model developed in the early twentieth century begins to explore the nature of consciousness for its own sake. Georges Gurdjieff, born in Armenia and trained in various Eastern traditions, taught a number of Sufi-based consciousness-altering techniques. He stated it in terms of identity states:

> "Every thought, every mood, every desire, every sensation, says 'I' ... Man's every thought and desire appears and lives quite separately and independently of the Whole. And the Whole never expresses itself.... Man is divided into a multiplicity of small I's." (quoted in Tart 1975, 165)

Gurdjieff's recommendation for understanding these various "I"s, or states of being, was self-observation, and he provided a wide range of tools for his students to use in that process. One of his students, P. D. Ouspensky, expanded on his teachings and methods through the 1940s and 1950s, linking them to the twentieth-century psychological models in his famous book, *In Search of the Miraculous.*

Students of esoteric psychology have developed a number of models to explain both the formation of patterns of mind functioning and the experiences that Tart has defined as Discrete States of Consciousness. Of these, perhaps the most widely read is Alice Bailey.

In *From Intellect to Intuition* (1932, 1974), Bailey identified five stages, or states, of consciousness to be achieved through the practice of *raja yoga* as she understood it. These are concentration, meditation, contemplation, illumination, and inspiration. Each of these states builds on the last, with meditation made possible by the experience of concentration, the depth of contemplation enabled by the experience of meditation, and so on. As did Gurdjieff, Bailey found that the path through these states is self-observation—both in stillness and in action.

Two classics of the field, Robert Ornstein's *Psychology of Consciousness* (1972) and Charles Hampden-Turner's *Maps of the Mind* (1982) were compilations of the many theories and models of mental functions that enabled the reader to place these ideas into some framework of distinctions and similarities. They provide an excellent overview of the many models that have been developed. Neither of them, however, provide a framework for working with the specific states of consciousness that we typically experience—and the others that we have the capacity to experience—in the course of our lives.

A wonderful exploration of consciousness observed is Itzhak Bentov's *Stalking the Wild Pendulum* (1977). Integrating the "hard sciences" of physics and chemistry with the "soft sciences" of psychology and anthropology, Bentov suggests that normal, waking consciousness is a small part of our total consciousness, pointing out that "in an altered state of consciousness we can expand our subjective time greatly" (ibid., 76). This corresponds with the findings of Robert Masters and Jean Houston, who provided guidelines for what they call "accelerated mental processes" in their classic handbook for guided meditation, *Mind Games* (1972). Bentov goes on to define a "state of being" as experiencing the totality of consciousness, or "the absolute" (Bentov 1977, 90). He suggests that meditation practices help us to achieve that "state of being" and so to integrate the various aspects and states of consciousness that we've experienced over our lives and also begin to sense the information and intelligence of other consciousnesses.

Depth of States and Opportunities for Development

As Tart continued to work with the states of consciousness reported in the literature and by his experimental subjects, he came to understand that within each state resided a range of potential experience. He noted that this range was not qualitative— was not a distinctly different quality, or state, of consciousness— but was, rather, a *quantitative* difference: a matter of more or less of the same qualities. He called this potential "depth" (1975, 182ff.).

Tart observed that as one goes deeper into a state of consciousness, the intensity of the qualities of that state tends to increase, until at a certain point—which varies by state—the intensity remains constant, while the depth may continue to increase. For example, one may be reading and reach a point where the internally generated images are clear and crisp while still being aware at some level of one's environment, and gradually become less and less aware of anything but the images associated with one's reading, although they are no more clear than before.

Tart's research, then, suggests that consciousness may be experienced in any one of many states, with greater or lesser depth or intensity in each state. We may develop our capacity to enter into different states at will, and to increase or decrease the depth and intensity of our experience in each state. Then, as we learn to experience increased depth in any particular state of consciousness, we experience increased ability to maintain the state and to prolong its effects on the mind-body system. This is why deep anxiety can lead to illness—and why deep meditation can lead to improved mind-body functioning well after the meditation period is completed.

Eastern Models

THE NATURE OF CONSCIOUSNESS has been the core study of Buddhist and Hindu *yogis* for more than a thousand years and a very refined set of concepts has evolved through the research, teachings, and literature of those traditions. Some of that literature was made available, in translation, as early as the mid-1800s, but it's only since the Tibetan diaspora that Westerners have had the opportunity to really study and comprehend the depth of the Buddhist model. Now, a number of books have been written in English to help facilitate the transfer of information.

Though there are several lineages of teaching, each with its own nuances and interpretation, they share some fundamental principles. *The Tibetan Book of Living and Dying* by Sogyal Rinpoche and *Glimpses of Abidharma* by Chögyam Trungpa Rinpoche are particularly useful in helping us understand these fundamentals.

In the Tibetan Buddhist model, there are two principles of human experience: *rigpa*, "pure awareness," free of any tendencies, free primordial wisdom; and alaya, "storehouse consciousness," the tendency to create all effects of karma, the tendency of mind to create life and death, the states known as samsara and nirvana, and the tendency to develop multiple kinds of consciousness. There are eight kinds of consciousness, usually listed as follows:

#1–5 are the five sense consciousnesses (seeing, smelling, hearing, tasting, and touching), understood as forms of projection, limited by

#6, the sixth sense, or "mind," which uses the five senses.

#7 can be called the unconscious and subconscious tendencies of mind.

#8 is the *alaya*, which breaks into the above tendencies dynamically through its creative energy. *Alaya* is Sanskrit; in Tibetan the word is *kunzhi* and means "the foundation of all things." It's the ground of all materiality, where karmic, or cause/effect, imprints are stored. It's the source of what Taoists call "the ten thousand things," or the material universe.

These eight consciousnesses are eight ways we project our beliefs and expectations onto the otherwise empty, or formless, void many times each minute. We project through the sense consciousnesses, through the "conscious mind," through the unconscious and sub-conscious tendencies. Through these projections we experience form, which we react to. This process creates further tendencies in us to react in similar ways, which is called *karma*.

However, what is called, in Tibetan, *rigpa* or *Dharmakaya* is most often spoken of as "the radiant ground of all existence," free of the limitations of form or feeling. Rigpa is awareness-itself. Psychologically it is open, spacious, and expansive in nature. *It is free of form and unaffected by karma.*

Since Buddhism emerged from Hinduism about 600 BCE, much of the language and many of the ideas are parallel. The ancient Sanskrit *Vedas* (5,000 to 8,000 years old) provide the basis for much of the Hindu model, expanded by the *Upanishads* (about a thousand years old) and codified in the *Yoga Sutras* of Patanjali, who is variously reported to have written anywhere from six hundred to sixteen hundred years ago. A number of translations of Patanjali's *Sutras* are available and a number of Hindu *yogis* have written English texts, helping us to understand the variations on the Hindu model. Perhaps the most famous of these is by Christopher Isherwood and Swami Prabhavananda, entitled *How to Know God* (1953), which is oriented toward the *Vedanta* school. Many later translations are available, but we will rely on Archie Bahm's *Yoga Sutras of Patanjali* (1961) for his simple and clear overview of the model.

Each of the several hundred *Sutras* is a statement that provides the basis for an interpretive reading or lecture. Patanjali's statements are the introductions to a series of lectures on the nature and practice of something that was referred to often in the ancient texts but never fully explained—hence the popularity of his work. (Bahm 1961, Introduction)

The practices of *yoga* are designed to free the self from any mental disturbance that might prevent union with the ultimate reality. These disturbances may be enjoyable or distressing, but all prevent the desired union.

Patanjali defines two kinds of consciousness. Bahm translates those as "normal consciousness ... occupied with investigating, distinguishing, enjoyment, and self-consciousness" (ibid., 44) and "superior consciousness" that "has freed itself from such occupation" (ibid., 45). He says that everyone may attain "superior consciousness" and that several factors contribute to the ease of that attainment, including one's natural tendencies, one's faith and commitment, and one's "wholehearted emulation of the Ideal Soul" (ibid., 51). "Ideal Soul" is Bahm's translation of the Sanskrit word *Ishwara*, which is often translated as "God." He points out that Patanjali's next *sutras* define the *Ishwara* in terms that are not consistent with the Western idea of God: "The Ideal Soul serves as the Supreme Example ... being timeless it exists at all times ... the traditional symbol 'OM' applies to it" (ibid., 54–55). Patanjali's next *sutra* recommends repetition of the "OM," with comprehension of its significance, as an aid in progressing toward superior consciousness—and Bahm reminds us that this "involves a giving of one's whole self to domination by attention to intonation of the universal, omnisonorous, self-contained meaning which it embodies" (ibid., 55).

As the *sutras* progress, Patanjali explains the various obstructions of normal consciousness and describes the various pitfalls one may encounter along the way. Then he begins to describe the experience of superior consciousness. "When one enjoys consciousness entirely freed from desire for results, then the true nature of all things becomes clear" (ibid., 75). Through the several hundred *sutras*, Patanjali explains how the mind and body are enhanced with the practice. Finally, in the summaries at the end of the series, Patan-jali tells us that "since the mind, freed from all its beclouding veils, enjoys a knowledge without limitations, there is nothing else left for it to [want to] know" (ibid., 157). In the final *sutra* we are told, "the soul, as pure awareness, remains perfectly pure" (ibid., 158).

Another *yoga* tradition, called *kriya* (from the roots *kri*, or "action," and *ya*, "awareness") *yoga*, and brought to the West by Paramahansa Yogananda, teaches that there are four states of consciousness:

1. physical consciousness: present during daily activities

2. dream consciousness: present during astral experiences or in waking mental activities

3. consciousness during deep sleep without dreams

4. pure consciousness: "*turiya*," . . . beyond the three others, their source, eternal, infinite without modification (Govindan 1991, 181)

Although this tradition is closely related to, and draws somewhat upon, the teachings of Patanjali, the focus is on the methods taught by Kriya Babaji Nagaraj as presented by Yogiar Ramaiah in Tamil Nadu, India, and Yogananda's teacher, Ishtewar. These involve pos-tures, movements, and visualization, as well as breath control. The ultimate goal of *kriya yoga* is to achieve a state of consciousness that is so much in union with the ultimate, so consistently *turiya*, that the body is transformed into "Effulgence of God" and disappears into light (ibid., 10).

Meditation, States of Consciousness, and Pure Awareness

WHEN MEDITATION METHODS were first introduced to West-erners there was a widely held belief that meditation was a particular state of consciousness. Bailey presented it as such in her stages, and even Tart described it as such in his early work (1969). Yet, although the ultimate goal of the meditation process may be to experience the state that Buddhists call *rigpa* or *samadhi*, Hindus call *turiya* or *nirvana*, and the Abramic traditions[11] call ecstatic Union with God, not all meditation methods achieve that end.

As research on the variety of meditation experiences continued, however, it became clear that meditation is not a unique state, but a means by which the individual can experience various levels of depth or intensity at any one of several states of consciousness— all of which may be located on the continuum of states described earlier in this chapter.

If we consider the many meditation methods available to us today, we can see that a range of depths, intensities, and states may be achieved. Some methods, like progressive neuromuscular release, shift our attention in a way that calms the mind-body system. Some, like focusing on a mantra or flame or flower, discipline the mind to concentrate and may begin to dissolve perceived boundaries between self and other. Some, like guided visualization or shamanic journeys, lead to an expanded perception of time, space, and the nature of reality. And so forth.

All of these methods, however, regardless of the depth or intensity or state of consciousness achieved, accomplish two things: they stop the habitual thought process and they restore a measure of harmony and resonance in the mind-body system so that its interacting patterns of thoughts, emotions, and physiological processes are no longer dysfunctional, but mutually supportive.

The Power of Pure Awareness

In his remarkable exploration into the nature of consciousness, Bentov suggests that

---

11. Judaism, Christianity, and Islam all honor the sacred writings that stem from "Father Abraham" and so are traditionally grouped together.

We can equate the state of being with the absolute, since both imply no motion, no action, and total rest. At the same time, though, it is a state of high potential energy, because this state of rest is infinitely fast motion ... tremendous energy and full of creative potential ... plus intelligence. This intelligence adds a self-organizing capability. (1977, 90)

His use of "state of being" is equivalent to the Buddhist concept of "pure awareness," both being "the absolute."

In the Buddhist tradition, *awareness* is characterized as having an intuitive, nonconceptual, direct knowing quality, timeless and unmoving. Mindfulness means being aware of mind and the activities of mind-body in living space. *Mind* is the constantly changing, self-centered conceptual activity intensely concerned with time, past and future. *Mind* is constantly talking and thinking about itself; *awareness* is open and free of self-preoccupation. *Mind* is most often not really focused on the present, tending to be involved with past and future. *Awareness* is always present; it's what people come home to when they shift attention out of the trances of mind back into living presence, where life is. *Awareness* is inborn, inherently free of mind. Though meditation science says that some aspects of *mind* probably derive from past-life experience, *mind* is predominantly a present-lifetime development, obscuring inherently free *awareness*. *Awareness* is continuously present as a free, unconditioned alternative to conditioned mind. The practice of intentional return to unconditioned *awareness* is a healthful release of unhealthy tendencies.

In distinguishing between mind and awareness it's essential to recognize two aspects of mind: *grasping* and *fixation*. Mind is developed through the interacting tendencies of grasping (attachment to objects) and fixation (attachment to self) *Grasping* is outwardly directed, attachment to the apparent phenomena of the world, defining the world in terms of one's own limited story. *Fixation* is inwardly directed attachment to the apparent subject of experience, "I," "me."

Through the process of observing our thoughts, we see that we fixate on ourselves because mind is afraid of losing itself, the believed subject of experience, often called "ego" or "small self." This tendency is called *zungwa* in Tibetan. As we observe further, we see that we hold on to external projections of a reality that is defined by the needs of the small self or ego to maintain itself— sometimes with such tenacity that we destroy our bodies and our relationships. This tendency is called *dzinpa* in Tibetan. The inter- actions of these tendencies form our thought processes and actions, which in turn limit and obstruct our capacity to simply be aware.

The Tibetan word *rigpa* is in Sanskrit *vidya*, which comes from a root meaning "to know, to understand, perceive, experience." Thus it can denote the action of knowing or understanding, with some emphasis on perceiving or seeing an object. And, at some lev- els of the meditative process, such "knowing" is experienced.

But at its deepest level there is no longer any separation between the seeing and the seen, the knowing and the known,[12] the medi- tator and the object of meditation. In the deepest state achieved through meditation one is resting in *rigpa*, free awareness, and not reacting to the eight kinds of tendency, thus breaking the karmic chain, the karmic pattern, and cutting off the unstable dynamic of form and action. In *rigpa* we return, in unmoving awareness, to the stable basis of health, the basis of psychological sanity, psycholog- ical health, and physiological homeostasis.

At the moment of the shift from *mind* back to *awareness, mind* attaches to that shift and is proud of itself, claiming to have made the shift. *Awareness* recognizes this tendency of mind, the tendency to fixation. *Awareness* is inherently free of that tendency and free of the shift back to itself. Both *mind* and the shift back to awareness

---

12. The Hebrew word *yada* (derived from the Sanskrit), which is usually translated as "to know" and sometimes refers to sexual intercourse, sug- gests the same idea of "union with," rather than "understanding of," that the Tibetan word *rigpa* suggests.

are discontinuous. *Awareness* is continuous. It has an unmoving, unchanging quality. *Awareness* is free of the practice of meditation. It is effortless. It is the basis for healing release.

Thus in *rigpa,* the experiences of psychological freedom, physical well-being, and panoramic awareness are inseparable. Pure awareness requires no energy to achieve or to sustain, and so the mind-body system can resume a balanced energy flow to and through the cells and organs. Pure awareness has no form or action, so the mind-body system can rest from response and reaction, allowing creative processes to resume and restore freely, without the limitations imposed by the need to respond.

This is why all the research into mind-body functioning of meditators shows high levels of functioning across the mind-body system. As we saw in Chapter Three, people who meditate regularly— almost regardless of meditation method—have better-than-average blood pressure, heart rate, hormone balances, immune function, muscle tone, cerebral functioning, recall, and comprehension.

Illness as a State of Consciousness

As WE CONSIDER THE CONTINUUM of states of consciousness in Figure 1 (p. 88), we see that some can be described as "more harmonious" and some as "less harmonious" with regard to the interacting functions of the mind-body system. For example, the states we've labeled Anxiety and Rage are associated with heightened adrenaline release, heart rate, and blood pressure—all of which disturb other physiological functions—and with limited mental functioning, which reduces the individual's capacity to respond to a changing environment. By contrast, in the state of Alert Rest the full range of mental function is operative and physiological functions are optimized.

To the extent that the experience of Illness is associated with physiological functions that are outside of normal, healthy functioning and to the extent that the person experiencing it is experiencing emotions of distress, Illness is clearly a "less harmonious" state of being. It's the state that results from ongoing dysfunctions in the mind-body system such that the body's normal responses to challenges are no longer sufficient to maintain healthy function. Therefore, to the extent that the body is perceived as the material manifestation of the particular thoughts, emotions, beliefs, and assumptions held by the individual at any given moment, Illness, indeed, must be understood as a state of consciousness.

Looking at Illness this way, we can identify a number of generic characteristics that apply almost regardless of the particular symptoms. The person experiencing the state of Illness:

- experiences body sensations acutely
- experiences challenges in multiple aspects of functioning
- has unique, more-frequent-than-normal periods of sleep and dreaming
- is more passive than active, and hence
- is freed from normal behavioral and reactive patterns

These characteristics apply to every experience of Illness, in whatever form. Indeed, they may be the defining characteristics of this particular state of consciousness.

This suggests, of course, that the way out of the experience of Illness is to change one's state of consciousness—exactly as Quimby, Eddy, Hopkins, and thousands of shamans and "faith healers" have done through the millennia (Miller 2000). They have treated the consciousness of the individual rather than the symptoms of the body. They have focused on restoring balance in the mind-body system rather than on "fixing" a particular structure or function in the body. As they have done so, the patient is transformed: she or he no longer functions in the same way.

Illness, then, like all states of consciousness, has its opportunities as well as challenges. Because of those opportunities, Illness may be understood as a process through which transformation becomes possible. With this book, we hope to identify the essential processes and methods that disclose the opportunities and make the inherent potential for transformation a reality.

References

Ashby, H. Ross. *An Introduction to Cybernetics*. New York: Pergamon, 1964.

Bahm, Archie. *Yoga Sutras of Patanjali*. Albuquerque, NM: University of New Mexico Press, 1961.

Bailey, Alice. *From Intellect to Intuition*. Wheaton, IL: Quest Books, 1932, 1974.

Bateson, Gregory. *Steps to an Ecology of Mind*. New York: Ballantine, 1972.

Bentov, Itzhak. *Stalking the Wild Pendulum*. Rochester, VT: Destiny Books, 1977.

Govindan, Marshall. *Babaji and the 18 Siddha Kriya Yoga Tradition*. Montreal: Kriya Yoga Publications, 1991.

Hampden-Turner, Charles. *Maps of the Mind*. New York: Macmillan, 1982.

Isherwood, Christopher, and Swami Prabhavananda. *How to Know God*. Los Angeles: Vedanta, 1953.

James, William. *The Varieties of Religious Experience*. New York: Doubleday & Co., 1978.

Jung, Carl G. *Memories, Dreams, Reflections*. New York: Vintage/Random House, 1965.

Masters, Robert, and Jean Houston. *Mind Games*. New York: Delta, 1972.

Miller, Ruth L. *150 Years of Healing*. Portland, OR: Abib, 2000.

Murphy, Michael. *The Future of the Body*. Los Angeles: Tarcher, 1992.

Murphy, Michael, and Steven Donovan. *The Physical and Psychological Effects of Meditation*. Sausalito, CA: IONS, 1999.

Ornstein, Robert. *Psychology of Consciousness*. New York: Viking, 1972.

Ouspensky, P. D. *In Search of the Miraculous*. New York: Harcourt, 1949.

Pearce, Joseph Chilton, and Thom Hartmann. *The Crack in the Cosmic Egg*. New York: Julian Press, 1971.

Sogyal Rinpoche. *The Tibetan Book of Living and Dying*. New York: HarperCollins, 1994.

Tart, Charles. *Altered States of Consciousness*. New York: Wiley, 1969.

———. *States of Consciousness*. New York: Dutton, 1975.

Trungpa, Chögyam. *Glimpses of Abidharma*. Boston: Shambhala, 1978.

CHAPTER 5

A New Model of the Body for a New Era of Medicine

THE SCIENTIFIC ADVANCES OF THE TWENTIETH and early twenty-first centuries have gone well beyond the model of human anatomy and function still adhered to by what Dr. Larry Dossey has called Era I, scientific-reductionist medicine. And, as we discovered earlier in this book, a number of Era II mind-body therapies have been demonstrated as effective healing methods within the Western scientific paradigm. These methods point to new understandings. Still, no comprehensive model of the dynamic nature of the human body has yet been presented to support these results and the ensuing shift to a new medical paradigm. Because we cannot present the therapeutic potential of the emerging medical paradigm without an appropriate vision of the human body, we will endeavor to present such an integrated model here.

An integrated model of the multidimensional human body appropriate for an expanded paradigm of medical science must

- be dynamic at every level
- take into consideration the vast range of interacting electromagnetic fields in the body that can be directly experienced as light
- offer explanations for therapies that work outside of the scientific-reductionist paradigm

Contributions to such a model must necessarily come from many disciplines, provided by ancient and contemporary scientists. We've drawn on the work of many researchers, from both modern and historically significant traditions. In addition, our model draws deeply from Tibetan science and its working knowledge of the energetic nature of the human body.

The Multiple Bodies of the Human Mind-Body

AS WE EXPLORE OUR USUAL EXPERIENCE of muscle, bone, and organs all packed into skin, and add our intuitive, imaginative, and emotional experience, we perceive several "bodies" to consider as our own. While this is not an understanding common in the Western scientific tradition, it is present in a number of other traditions.

The Western Spiritual Model

Although the religious traditions of the West have not been built on a psychology of consciousness, there are elements of a multi-body model of human experience expressed in both the sacred literature and daily practice of Judaism, Christianity, and Islam (the Abramic traditions) that should not be ignored in our search for a working model of the mind-body.

Within these traditions each individual consists of a soul and a body and is isolated from all others except God. The body is considered to be the physical and emotional manifestation, experiences, and expressions of the individual. The soul, while not fully integrated with the body, is understood to be the life force of the body and is affected by the body's experiences and expressions—its destiny being determined, in large part, by them. This split between the body and the soul is fundamental to the practices and principles of all three traditions, is what permits Muslim "suicide bombers" to feel good about what they do, and is what drove the Catholic Church to "save souls" without regard to the state of the body for so many years.[13]

A third element, called Spirit, enters into the picture with the New Testament. It originally referred to what Jesus called "the Comforter" and was experienced as a wind and a flame at Pentecost. The apostle Paul, exhorting his followers not to "walk in the way of the flesh" but of Spirit (Romans 7 and 8 et al.) and encouraging them to develop "gifts of the Spirit" (I Corinthians et al.), shifted the original concept from an experience to a state of being. The current idea is that, through God's good grace and no effort or special deserving, "the Holy Spirit enters in" to some people and transforms them, providing gifts such as prophecy and healing. It's a central element of the Pentecostal Christian movement, charismatic Catholicism, and many of the fundamentalist Protestant doctrines. In metaphysical New Thought churches, the Holy Spirit is understood to be the omnipresent essence of all that is, formless yet expressing through and as each being.

The "Christ mind," which Paul exhorted his followers to "let be in your mind" (Philippians 2) adds another dimension to the model. He defined this mind as a way of being that exhibits no human emotion or judgment, offering only compassion, unconditional love, and acceptance. In the metaphysical New Thought churches, this is considered a state of consciousness, called Christ Consciousness, that can be attained through prayer, meditation, and affirmation.

The model becomes somewhat blurred with the integration of "spiritualist" Judaism and Christianity into the picture. In this tradition, Jesus and the prophets are understood to have conversed

---

13. One of the miracles of Mother Teresa's work was that she persuaded the Roman Catholic Church to allow her to focus on tending the dying bodies of the "unsaved"—not as a means to save them, but because they were, in her eyes, the embodiment of Christ.

with people who have "passed on" and are no longer in physical form (for example, the disciples' observation of Jesus' conversation with Moses and Elijah in the story called "The Transfiguration"), and so modeled for their followers that they should do likewise. Spiritualist churches therefore include channeling of messages from "the other side" in their otherwise traditional Christian services, and what is known as "voodoo" includes many such activities in otherwise Christian services. This practice introduced the idea of the individual spirit into the cultural conversation, which is sometimes confused with the biblical concept of soul, because both exist before and after this lifetime.

In the mid-nineteenth century, with the first translations of sacred texts from the East, a new model emerged within the Christian tradition as part of the Transcendentalist movement. Ralph Waldo Emerson, Henry David Thoreau, Walt Whitman, Margaret Fuller, and the Alcotts were instrumental in bringing into popular American awareness the fundamental ideas of this movement. These include: the possibility of a direct perception of reality, unmediated by thought; a unification with mankind and Nature; an identification with the divine as Oversoul; and a way of being that transcends social norms and expectations. One significant development out of this movement was the application of these ideas in the form of Christian Science and the New Thought tradition. Both Christian Science and New Thought see the body as the manifestation of all of the thoughts, beliefs, ideas, and expectations held in mind, the individual mind as a part of a universal Mind of God, and the individual soul or spirit as part of the eternal, omnipresent Spirit of God (Miller 2000).

The Western Esoteric Model

A large body of literature has emerged over the past two centuries attempting to explain the human experiences that the materialist-scientific tradition can't, and traditional religion has not been willing to, explain. Pollsters call these experiences "mystical" and poll results over the past several decades range from around 50 percent to more than 80 percent of Americans acknowledging having them. (This will not surprise regular listeners of the popular nighttime radio talk show *Coast to Coast AM*.) Some of the reported experiences include seeing "ghosts" and feeling, smelling, or hearing invisible presences; seeing or hearing a nonmaterial being acting to guard or protect one; observing things or beings appear or disappear in inexplicable ways; unexplained healings and remissions of disease; and direct visual or oral communications with people who are known to be elsewhere.

The lack of religious or scientific explanations for these experiences in the nineteenth and early twentieth centuries led scientifically minded folks to rigorously investigate such experiences, which in turn led to the formation of the British Society for Psychical Research, the Theosophical Society, and several other associations seeking to understand scientifically what was explained by neither science nor religion. The reports of rigorous tests in the journals and books produced by these associations and their members are numerous and exhaustive.

One summary of these texts is *The Basic Ideas of Occult Wisdom* by Anne Kennedy Winner (1970). She says:

> We are told that every human body, besides the dense physical core which we see, has in it and around it a number of interpenetrating sheaths (sheath in the sense of container, as a possible container of the spirit), each made up of the world of the ... subtle worlds.... every man has an "etheric" or "vital" sheath or body, which is physical in the sense of belonging to the physical plane, and in being discarded at death, but which is invisible to ordinary sight, because it is made up of "matter" of the finest or "etheric" subdivisions of the physical plane ... a kind of "force field" which forms the matrix or energy pattern upon which the dense physical form is built ... (35)

In *The Doctrine of the Subtle Body in Western Tradition*, G. R. S. Mead explores the various understandings of spirit, ethereal body, subtle body, and related concepts throughout Western history (1919, 1967). Drawing on the writings of minds as diverse as Plato and Tertullian, Aristotle and Menander, Mead summarizes dozens of conceptualizations of the human being as consisting of something more than a material body, having something variously termed a "spirit," a "subtle body," a "soul," and a "resurrection body." Together, these writings point to a model of the human being in which an eternal essence takes form in two stages: as spirit or subtle body and then as material body. Then, through imagination, thought, word, and activity, the two together facilitate the subtle body's return to the eternal, and the material body is either discarded or resurrected in union with the spirit.

In *Vibrational Medicine* (1988), Richard Gerber, MD, integrates a model of human function that describes five inseparable bodies: the physical body, a mental body, an astral body, an etheric body, and a causal body. This multifold body model permits different levels and types of activity and explains the different types of human experience.

According to Gerber, the physical body is the material, manifest body that interacts with the material world around it. The mental body is the field of energy that is formed by and forms one's thoughts and logical reasoning and so affects the functioning of the material body. The astral body is composed of a substance that is neither matter nor energy and so is not limited by the laws of matter, but can function in the material world as well as on what is called "the astral plane," a dimension of existence that is very dreamlike and is, according to many, where much of our dreamwork happens. (Being built on emotions and irrational feelings, the astral body has a profound impact on the material body and is the body-form of most "ghosts"—beings whose life experiences were so intense that they have been unable to leave the situation of the experiences.) The etheric body is almost pure energy and corresponds to the unique self, or spirit, of the individual. Like the astral body, it transcends space and time, but it is pure awareness, free of the intense emotions that drive and form the astral body. The causal body is that aspect of self that experiences this lifetime as part of an eternal experience and carries into this lifetime memories and understandings from other lifetimes. It is sometimes referred to as the Higher Self.

> The etheric and physical bodies, being of different frequencies, overlap and coexist within the same space.... Energy disturbances in the etheric body and the acupuncture meridian system precede the physical/cellular manifestation of illness.... The astral body is ... made up of matter of a higher frequency than etheric matter. It is similarly superimposed upon the physical-etheric framework.... Consciousness can move into the astral body and separate from the physical-etheric vehicles. When this occurs naturally it is known as astral projection of an Out-Of-Body Experience (OOBE). When this separation of consciousness occurs traumatically it is often referred to as a Near Death Experience (NDE)....
> (Gerber 1988, 171–72)

Every moment of human existence, in this model, is experienced through the interaction of these bodies. Individual development, therefore, is seen as the capacity to identify and choose which body one is operating from at any time—gradually moving from the physical and astral through the mental to the causal and etheric, or eternal/celestial essence. Ultimately, one aims to be aware of all of them all the time and to act in ways that ensure harmony at all levels.

The Three-Part Buddhist Model

The Buddhist description of the *trikaya*, literally meaning "the three bodies," offers another compelling model of the multidimensional nature of humanity. Having emerged from the *Vedic* tradition, the

Buddhists use Sanskrit terms for these aspects of being: *Dharmakaya,*
Sambhogakaya, and *Nirmanakaya.* Francesca Fremantle, in her book
Luminous Emptiness, describes the *trikaya* as "the threefold pattern
of the awakened state," stating that Chögyam Trungpa Rinpoche
used to speak of it as the pattern of life in general.

Dharmakaya means "truth body" or "body of absolute nature."
Psychologically this is defined as the empty or open nature of the
body, inseparable from pure awareness. It can be defined as the
quantum field within the atomic nature of the corporal form, the
subatomic void of pure potential, from which the universe and its
infinite forms emerge. The *Dharmakaya* is the nonlocal, universal
field, the basis of the being's unlimited nature, its timeless, deathless nature (referred to in Dossey 1999). The *Dharmakaya* corresponds
to what Georges Gurdjieff referred to as *essence,* the fundamental
nature of the being; it is what physicist Amit Goswami (1993) calls
the consciousness that pervades and creates the material world.

Spontaneously arising from the *Dharmakaya* is the *Sambhogakaya,*
which is the connecting form, the body of light, the body of communication. Fremantle describes it in terms of light:

> Light radiates from the emptiness of dharmakaya as the five
> colors of the five kinds of knowledge. It appears in shining
> rainbow clouds, in glowing circles, in scintillating pinpoints,
> and dazzling rays of light. Then the five colors crystallize
> into ... divine forms ... made entirely of light; they arise out
> of light and dissolve back into light. This is the realm of sacred
> vision ... the bridge between emptiness and form: emptiness
> displaying itself as form; form revealing itself to be empti-
> ness. (2001, 178)

In Buddhist meditation *Sambhogakaya* is the visionary form of
the various aspects of deity nature, a radiant form within the material body. Visualizing this form can be understood as a practice of
seeing the divine energy body as the body of our potential. As Fremantle puts it,

The experience of the sambhogakaya is to perceive the world directly and nakedly, welcoming whatever appears without preconceptions. Sense perceptions become clearer, sharper, and more colorful.... The world is recognized as sacred, magical, and full of wonder. It contains all the vitality and passion of the emotions, free from the confusion that brings misery and pain. (ibid.)

One focuses on this radiant "bridge between emptiness and form," this inner light, in order to:

- communicate with the unlimited potential of the *Dharmakaya* within
- practice the wisdom and power of the light nature of embodiment, the *Sambhogakaya*, radiating well-being into all aspects of being
- not lose our true nature by identifying only with the manifest nature, the *Nirmanakaya*
- restore balance and set body, mind, and spirit in primal order
- thus restore health and access our inherent potential

The *Nirmanakaya*, or manifest nature, is the actual physical manifestation: energy appearing as matter to act in the realm of matter. The term literally means "body of emanation," because it emanates from the *Sambhogakaya*. It is sometimes called "the causal body." In its highest form, it is the embodiment of the energy of compassion and totally responsive to the needs of all beings; the Tibetan term for this highest form is *tulku*, a title given to one who is recognized as a great teacher reborn with full awareness of his or her buddha-nature and with the conscious intention to benefit others. However, as Fremantle reminds us, "we are all really nirmanakaya, but we do not realize it" (ibid., 180).

The Buddhist model, therefore, places the material body in a matrix of universality *(Dharmakaya)* and radiant divinity *(Sambhogakaya)*, through which it emerges as an expression and experience of both. With this model, all of life's processes can be seen as movement within and among these three aspects of being, and focusing on the radiant light nature of the *Sambhogakaya* becomes a means for bringing a higher order of functioning to them all. Fremantle says:

> The experience of the trikaya can be found everywhere; it is a continual presence in our lives. The dharmakaya is present in the sense of openness, the source and background of all phenomena. The sambhogakaya is present in the sense of energy bursting forth, the sacred, magical quality of life. And the nirmanakaya is present in the sense of phenomena continually arising, impermanent yet vividly apparent. (ibid., 75)

Within this threefold structure, Buddhist research says that each sentient being has three "doors"—body, speech, and mind— through which our deeds, thoughts, and words work in the world. Body refers to the manifest, material form and corresponds to the *Nirmanakaya*. "It is the outward expression in material form of our mind and energy" (ibid., 180). Speech corresponds to *Sambhogakaya*: energy, emotion, and communication. It refers to both the outward sounds and the inner emotions from which they emanate. The invisible, formless mind corresponds to the *Dharmakaya*, including all our thoughts, perceptions, feelings, and reactions, and encompassing the Western ideas of heart and mind, together.

Fremantle points out that the same tri-fold pattern continues in the Buddhist concept of "coarse, subtle, and very subtle body and mind" saying that these three correspond to "the waking state, the state of dreaming, and the state of deep sleep" (ibid., 185). The coarse body is the flesh-and-blood-and-bones that we usually think of as our body, including the hormonal and nerve systems that manifest specific states, and corresponds to the *Nirmanakaya*. The subtle body, or mind-body, like the *Sambhogakaya*, bridges between our physical experience and pure awareness in the dream state. The

very subtle body is nearly indescribable, corresponding to the emptiness of the *Dharmakaya*, typically illustrated as the union of the male
and female principles in the heart. It is often called the intrinsic
buddha-nature and is the essence of life, "a continuity of luminous
awareness" (ibid., 193).

The Upanishads

Perhaps the most ancient documented scientific research may be
found in the Hindu *Upanishads*, written in Sanskrit somewhere
between 5,000 and 8,000 years ago. Buddhist researchers knew the
models presented in these ancient texts and incorporated many of
the concepts into their own frameworks.

One of these is the idea of a subtle body overlapping the physical body, with a threefold nature, described in Sanskrit: *nadi, prana,*
and *bindu*. In this model, *nadi*, which means "tube" or "channel,"
refers to a network of energy channels that form the structure of
the subtle or energy body. Like the network of acupuncture points
recognized in Chinese medicine, the network of *nadis* can be imagined as tubes through which life energy flows, sustaining the physical body.

This energy is called *prana*, which can be translated as "energy,"
"spirit," "life," or "breath." Like the Greek *pneuma*, which also translates as both "spirit" and "breath," *prana* can be experienced in the
air around us, available through breathing, and in our bodies,
enlivening our cells.

In the Upanishads this pranic level of being is described as
... a second body within the physical body called the "vital
body" or "vital sheath." ... the physical body is nothing more
than a crystallization around the energy pattern that underlies it. (Rama 1979, 10, 13)

The creative impulse for this network is the *bindu*, which is
described by Fremantle as "the seed point that contains the whole

of existence and spreads out infinitely to pervade and encompass the expanse of space" (2001, 263). She says it is

... the basic nature of our mind and the essence of life, a continuity of luminous awareness. (ibid., 193)

Mind and bindu are very closely related, with bindu as the basis or instigator of all the different kinds of consciousness. Mind is the creator of everything ... but bindu is the creative spark ... Mind or consciousness observes, watches what is going on, and responds to it. Bindus pervade the subtle body; they are carried around by prana and they gather in the chakras where they cause the different modes of consciousness to arise. (ibid., 190)

This concept of *bindu* as seed point, or seed essence, is also the sexual essence in men and women. It is, in Tibetan, translated as *thigle*, which is described in some detail later in this book.

The subtle or energy body described by the *Upanishads* explains much of our internal experience and has provided the basis for many of the healing practices of Hindu and Buddhist cultures.

Energy Body Channels

The subject of energy body anatomy has been in the public domain since the publication of *The Anatomy of the Spirit* by Caroline Myss (1994) and has been offered by teachers of various meditation science traditions since the 1970s.

In Myss' popular presentation, a series of power centers, or *chakras*, are aligned along a central energy channel that begins at the anus and rises to the crown *chakra*. She combines this model with other understandings of the body as a map for intuitive appreciation of the energy dynamics of the individual.

In *Vibrational Medicine* Gerber states that there is

... considerable evidence to suggest that there exists a holographic energy template associated with the physical body ... [within which] information is carried which guides the cellular growth of the physical structure of the body ... There are specific channels of energy exchange which allow the flow of energetic information to move from one system to another. (1988, 121)

The ancient teachings of Indo-Tibetan meditation science describe a body of at least 72,000 major and minor energy channels, with equally extensive systems of associated subtle channels, which come into and go out of existence quickly in the mass dynamic of the whole energy body system. For present purposes, we will focus on the larger, more obvious features of the energy body and its characteristics in relation to the physical body.

The *chakra* model comes from the Sanskrit *Vedas*. In this understanding, the central energy channel, with its vertical series of *chakras* or energy power centers, corresponds with the central nervous system and with glands of the endocrine system. For instance, the *crown chakra* is traditionally associated with the cerebral cortex, while the "third eye" *chakra* is associated with the pineal gland and hypothalamus. For a more complete description of the *chakras* and their correspondences in the nervous and endocrine systems we refer the reader to Myss (1994) or Gerber (1988). Here we are concerned in general with the energy body features and their effects on the overall physical systems.

Beyond their correspondence with aspects of the nervous and endocrine systems, the *chakras*, or dynamic energy wheels, are vortices of subtle energies

... somehow involved in taking in higher [frequency] energies and transmuting them to a utilizable form within the human structure ... From a physiologic standpoint, the *chakras* appear to be involved with the flow of higher energies via specific subtle energetic channels into the cellular structure of the human body. At one level they seem to function as transformers, stepping down energy of one form and frequency to a lower energetic level. (Gerber 1988, 128)

This energy is in turn transmuted into neural and hormonal changes on a cellular level throughout the body through the series of energy channels called, in Sanskrit, *nadis,* and recognized by acupuncturists as energy meridians. Through centuries of experience Tibetan masters have verified all the dimensions of the energy body and its integral relation to the physical body that were described in those ancient texts. They've found that there are subtle aspects of the nervous and endocrine systems that may be observed for the first time in subtle but well-defined aspects of the energy body system and that have correspondences with physical systems. A Western doctor, Dharma Singh Khalsa, MD, observes that these correspondences have been

> ... verified by the use of sophisticated radioactive scanning methods. The *nadis* are formed by fine threads of subtle energetic matter ... *Nadis* are an extensive network of fluid-like [energy ducts] which parallel the body nerves in their abundance. The *nadis* are interwoven with the physical energy system—in intricate interconnection—affecting the nature and quality of nerve transmission within the extensive network of the central nervous system. (Khalsa 2001, 131)

The central energy channel is most often spoken of in its association with two parallel "side channels," making up three main energy channels.

> The three main *nadis* are connected to the brain's limbic system, which controls memory and emotion. It also coordinates the functions of the hypothalamus, and helps control the endocrine's master gland, the pituitary. The [energy body has] a tremendously important effect on the body's biochemistry. (ibid., 23)

Disturbance of the structure of, or dysfunction in, the *chakras* and *nadis*, or acupuncture meridians, precedes and is associated with pathological changes in the nervous and endocrine systems. Such dysfunction can result in quantitative and qualitative dysfunction of the subtle energetic flow to the physical substance and, via the hormonal link, can create abnormalities in the body.

> The *nadis* appear to physically affect the nature and quality of nerve transmission from the brain and spinal cord to the outlying peripheral nerves. Therefore energy blockage among the *nadis* seems to be associated with the closely associated endocrine and immune systems. For example, a decreased flow of energy through the *nadis* to the throat *chakra* might result in decreased energy to the thyroid. The physical manifestation of this might be hypothyroidism. (ibid., 23)

Long-proven methods such as *Bum Chung* (Vase Breathing) access both the energy and physical systems at once. As described by G. C. C. Chang, *Bum Chung* brings in vital energy, through breathing *prana* into the central channel, simultaneously with shifting from mind to the energetic field of awareness (Chang 1963, 57–60).

The Energetic Mind-Body

A S WE LOOK AT THE IDEAS that emerged in the twentieth-century sciences, we discover a new set of understandings about the nature of matter and the human mind-body system.

Fields Within Fields

In current scientific understanding, atoms and molecules are seen not as solid structures but as a dynamic result of the interactions of fields of the greatest forces of the universe. Instead of solid particles rotating around each other like planets and suns, atoms are now known to be largely open space, with "clouds" or "fields" of positive and negative energy interacting in a cosmic balancing act.[14] It was this understanding that led Deepak Chopra to write *Quantum Healing*.

This new perspective gives us a human body that looks far more like a set of constantly changing interactive fields than anything fixed or solid. The ongoing quantum-mechanical activity can be understood as patterns of vibration, sometimes in the particle-form of matter and sometimes in the wave-form of energy. In particle-form, the atomic substance of which we are composed is located in a particular point of space and time, with the density of matter. In wave-form, the same substance cannot be located, because it's everywhere in space and time.

> ... an atom ... occupies two distinct states, so many times a second ... Our matter is blinking on and off ... constituted by a rapid succession of instantaneous events ... Our bodies are oscillators ... we expand into a spacelike dimension many times a second ... and collapse back as rapidly. (Bentov 1977, 56, 76)

Energy, being the wave-form of subatomic substance, is not fixed in time and space. When an atom is split, the part of it that becomes energy is everywhere immediately, which is why the results of subatomic experiments are so strongly affected by the way the experiment was structured—there is no past, present, or distance for energy at the subatomic level.[15]

---

14. A number of filmmakers have done an excellent job of portraying this new understanding of the nature of matter. Brian Greene's *The Elegant Universe*, available through PBS, and *What the BLEEP Do We Know!?* are particularly effective.

15. For some interesting, readable explanations of this phenomenon, try Danah Zohar, *The Quantum Self*, Amit Goswami's *The Self-Aware Universe*, or anything by Fred Alan Wolf.

Though it is often portrayed as something like the rings of water that emanate from a pebble striking the surface of a pond, energy is not *moving across* space, but rather *fills* space—in all directions. We turn on a light and it fills the room; we light a fire and the heat fills the flame, every which way. The light, the heat, the electricity—all are *fields* of energy.

The same is true with the energy of our bodies. It exists as fields, only partially contained within the bone and tissue. This means that the fields of energy that we are can't be seen as limited to the material body. Like all fields of energy, the fields of energy that we are can't be limited by space or time. And the fields of energy that we are interact to create a variety of new, resonating patterns of possibility.

Advances in technology and an emerging body of research in the electromagnetic nature of the human body have shown that the body's biomagnetic field effects extend into space without obstruction. The heart beat and all the muscles in the body produce electromagnetic fields, active inside the body and in space. The body's vibrations and oscillations act in many frequencies, internally and externally.

> Every muscle in the body produces magnetic pulses when it contracts. The large muscles produce larger fields and the smaller muscles, such as those that move and focus the eye, produce very tiny fields ... The fields of all the organs spread throughout the body and into the space around it. (Oschman 2000, 35–37)

The stability of these fields is a function of the rhythms—the patterns of vibration—they share. Dr. Karl Maret, one of the researchers exploring these new perceptions, has found that

> All living processes in the body depend on the transfer of charges to conduct energy and support life. The entire watery matrix of our bodies is interconnected by complex charge-coupled fields that receive about sixty pulsations of electro-

magnetic energy from our beating heart each minute.... Every cell in the body is in intimate electromagnetic contact with the toroidal-shaped magnetic field of the heart. (Maret, in Oschman 2000, x)

The balancing act of multiple forces moderated by a single organ, the heart, results in an appearance of constancy and continuity in the mind-body.

We can see these patterns in electroencephalograms (EEGs), in electrocardiograms (EKGs), and in magnetic resonance imaging scanners (MRIs). As we have seen, the oscillating fields that make up our body shift from the density of matter to the infinity of energy many times each second as the atomic substance that makes up each field oscillates in a particular pattern of vibration: particle/matter–wave/energy, and back again. The particular set of interacting fields that we are has a particular pattern of oscillation, so we each have a unique resonating pattern of possibility.

In the process, as it encounters other energy forms, the pattern of our bodies is easily influenced, yet remarkably stable.

Our biological rhythms are entrained by light and to a certain extent by gravitational effects ... magnetic, electromagnetic, atmospheric, and subtle geophysical effects influence us.... Our mind-body is resonant with these rhythmically entrained field effects, natural and man-made. We're also surrounded and permeated by the static electricity field and by the electrostatic fields created by our body. (Bentov 1977, 30)

Thus, as opposed to the historical conceptualization of the body as a set of replaceable material-mechanical structures, the human body is now most fundamentally understood as a set of interacting universal fields of energy, operating across the electromagnetic spectrum.

James Oschman expresses this beautifully in *Energy Medicine: The Scientific Basis:*

On the basis of what is now known about the roles of electrical, magnetic, elastic, acoustic, thermal, gravitational, and photonic energies in human systems, it appears that there is no single "life force" or "healing energy" in living systems. Instead there are many energetic systems in the living body, and many ways of influencing those systems, both known and unknown, functioning collectively, cooperatively, synergistically. The debate about whether there is such a thing as a healing energy or life force is being replaced with the study of the interactions between biological energy fields, structures and functions. (Oschman 2000, 219)

Interestingly, this understanding, while the result of the most modern physical and biophysical investigation, is also an ancient one, with variations in cultures ranging from Tibet to Mexico, Siberia to Australia. For example, in *The Active Side of Infinity*, a Yaqui shaman shared the ancient teachings of this tradition by asserting that

... when a human being was *seen*, he was perceived as a conglomerate of energy fields held together by the most mysterious force in the universe: a binding, agglutinating, vibratory force that holds energy fields together in a cohesive unit. (Castaneda 1998, 70)

An understanding of the human body as essentially energetic is also the basis for a number of traditional and increasingly well-known healing modalities, perhaps the most familiar of which is the ancient Chinese practice of acupuncture and its close relative, acupressure.

So, in physics and in mysticism, matter and energy are no longer seen as separate substances, but as different ways of perceiving the same thing. More and more, Westerners are discovering that our experience of the body as static matter is simply a function of our conditioning. The shamanic traditions and higher initiations of many cultures lead individuals who are open to the mystery of transcendent reality into a new experience of the body, giving them, as Carlos Castaneda described above, the ability to see people, animals, and plants as interacting fields of energy. It was the discovery of this understanding in the mystical traditions that led physicist Fritjof Capra to write his seminal work, *The Tao of Physics,* launched the work of Ken Wilber, and inspired the movie, *What the BLEEP Do We Know!?*

Universal Energy Sustaining the Body

Whereas Western science has not yet developed a model for the exchange of energy that sustains the energy system of the body, Eastern traditions offer rich explanations.

> When you breathe, you don't just breathe in a gaseous mixture containing oxygen. You also breathe in *prana,* the universal life force. The ancient *yoga* masters were far more interested in the ethereal aspect of breathing than in the obvious physical aspect. (Khalsa 2001, 55)

What are the energies that can be breathed?

The life-energy of the universe, the energy that the Nobel Prize–winning biochemist Ilya Prigogine (1984) found essential for maintaining living systems, is called *prana* or *chi* in the Eastern meditation sciences in which it is most frequently used.

Traditionally this energy is differentiated into internal and external *chi* or *prana.* (In the previous section we explored its use, describing an aspect of the subtle body in the *Upanishads.*) The Taiwanese researcher Pei-Chen Lo suggests that the internal *chi* is different from the absolute energy of the universe (Lo, Huang, and Chang 2003). Most traditions, however, describe both forms as the same "vital force," permeating all matter.

Perennial wisdom says *prana* is the vital force that is the difference between animate and inanimate objects. *Prana* is omnipresent and universal, the power generating life. *Prana* is vital energy alive in the air. Meditation science says that *prana* can be experienced and breathed without using the senses. When people transmit "heal-ing energy," *prana* may be the energy transmitted.

In Tibetan, the translation of *prana* is *lung*, which is air, or wind, or psychic energy. The word inspiration literally means "to breathe in." The Greek word for breath, *pneuma*, also means "soul" or "spirit." The Japanese word for the universal energy, *Ki*, also means air. In Chinese, the fundamental universal energy field is called *chi*, like the life force *chi* of the living body, and it is usually referred to as the same thing.

It's because of the natural affinity of the *prana* of the "external" universal/quantum field for the *prana* of the human body, in the "internal" quantum field, that *prana* is breathable. This fundamen-tal vital energy is in the air, different from air and one with air at the same time. It can be sensed and breathed. In *kriya yoga, prana* is understood as the "nerve force" without which

> the heart cannot beat, the lungs cannot breathe; the blood cannot circulate and the various organs cannot perform their respective normal functions. This *prana* not only supplies electric force to the nerves, but it also magnetizes the iron in the system and produces the *aura* as a natural emanation.... the student of yogic breathing can actually feel the flow of energy throughout the network of nadis during each breath. (Govindan 1991, 154, 156)

Tibetan *Vajrayana* meditation practitioners learn to breathe, absorb, and optimize the functioning of the five airs, or forms of *lung*, flowing in the subtle energy channels of the manifest body. *Vajrayana* Buddhism, like Hindu meditation science, identifies five kinds of *lung* functioning in the body. It also discerns five kinds of energy operating in the phenomenal world. The five internal *pranas* that *Vajrayana* Buddhism considers integral to the function of the human body are:

- all-pervading in the body
- circulating upward
- preventing deterioration
- holding life force
- circulating downward

This understanding is a small fragment of a substantial, mostly unpublished knowledge-base transmitted from teacher to student and is described more fully in the Appendix. It is taught as part of learning to breathe the *prana* energy into the Life Vase *(Tse Bum)*, intentionally enhancing the functioning of the five *lungs* or *pranas* in the body. It is the basis for the method described later in this book as awareness-based energy breathing.

In terms of Western science, what is *lung/prana/chi*? Clearly, it is the energy that Prigogine describes as essential for maintaining the integrity of any living system. Yet we could say it is not truly either energy or matter; rather, it may be the essence of the quantum field, from which all matter and energy arise. It can be described as "matter on the verge of becoming energy or energy on the point of becoming matter" (Kaptchuk 1983, 35) and is sometimes referred to as the Universal Energy Field (UEF) (Brennan 1990, 63). It is the subtle energy from which all matter evolves, the energy of the void of the absolute potential from which the world emerges, which remains inseparable from the emergent matter. It is, in the literature of Buddhist meditation science, *Dharmakaya*, the energetic void that is the potential of all life and emerges in bond with all life (Dudjom 2001, 89; Thinley Norbu 1985, 66; Longchen Rabjam 1989, 200–212ff.).

Light in the Body

The substance of the universe, the "quantum field of potential," can be understood as a matrix out of which subatomic units sometimes show up as waves of energy and sometimes as particles of matter. These units have been called "wavicles" by quantum physicists and they interact in patterns of vibration that we perceive as the universe—and our bodies.

The most common of these wavicles is the photon, the basic unit of light, which in normal life we experience as sometimes showing up as a laser beam or as a ray or field of light, and sometimes as a particle hitting, for instance, a computer or television screen. And, as the structures that make up the human body are analyzed and understood using today's technologies, it becomes clear that living cells, tissue, and organs appear to generate, and possibly communicate through, light fields and beams—along with other electrochemical signals and fields.

Quantum physicist Herbert Frölich demonstrated in the 1970s that living tissue, when "pumped up" with high levels of energy, emits electromagnetic vibrations, or photons.

> From the work of Frölich and others, we now know that all parts of the living matrix set up vibrations that move about within the organism, and that are radiated into the environment. These vibrations or oscillations occur at many different frequencies, including visible and near visible light ... (Oschman 2000, 62)

Again, this concept is not new. The philosophical and healing traditions of many cultures, including Western Judeo-Christian literature, have suggested it for several thousand years. In Judeo-Christian traditions, light is synonymous with wisdom, life, and divine power. In Buddhism our fundamental nature is known to be "clear light." It is our potential. What is "clear light"? Revered Buddhist texts say that it's the radiant luminosity of the ground of being, and it's obstructed by ordinary consciousness. It's revealed the moment before death, when the tendencies of this lifetime have all dissolved. According to these texts, the great luminosity of the basis of life is revealed to everyone at that time. If they have practiced meditation during their lifetime they will, to some degree, recognize the clear light as their own nature. Otherwise it isn't recognized (Sogyal 1994, 263–65). The clear light may also manifest in orgasm, and sometimes in sneezing, but it's rarely recognized (Fremantle 2001, 193).

Dr. Pei-Chen Lo, of the National Chiao Tung University in Taiwan, decided to test the validity of these ancient references. Studying Zen meditation practitioners, using the electroencephalogram (EEG), he found that

> Zen-Buddhist practitioners have discovered that the *inner energy* is the resource of health and bliss. According to our investigation, the practitioners through years of Zen-Buddhist practice can change the constitution of their bodies by igniting the inner energy. A large number of practitioners are found not only to maintain better health but to remain younger and more energetic than normal people do. (Lo, Huang, and Chang 2003, 620)

Lo distinguishes the energy of "spiritual *chi*" from "inner light," suggesting that "the spiritual *chi* can be transformed, via orthodox Zen Buddhist meditation practice, into electrical *chi* and even light *chi* that is finally the light of eternal life" (ibid.). He concludes that the more someone experiences his or her inner light, through training and practice, the more he or she will experience enhanced health.

Mind-Body Energy in Context

We have established that the body is a unique set of interactive energy fields within a larger field of interactive fields that, ultimately, surround the Earth. These fields are measurable on the electromagnetic spectrum and their activity is observed through a variety of technologies.

The effects on the body of the electromagnetic fields around the Earth can be understood in two ways. One effect is simple: the Earth's composite field, though made of energy and information, works a little like gelatin. When our mind-bodies move and vibrate, these movements are transmitted into the larger field. So, just as a movement in one part of a gelatin dessert can be seen to cause the rest of the gelatin in the dish to move, what we do affects the whole field. Conversely, other people's movements in the field affect our mind-bodies and the electrical charges of specific nerves and chemicals inside our bodies. These, in turn, affect cellular function. As cellular biologist Bruce Lipton has demonstrated, the receptors on the cell membrane will act as if a chemical is present *even if only the electrical pattern of that chemical* is present. These receptors, in turn, direct the cell's activities (Lipton 2005).

The electromagnetic fields around the Earth affect us in other ways, too. Our planet is surrounded by a moving layer of electrically charged particles called the ionosphere. The Earth being made up of water and minerals that are predominantly negatively charged and the ionosphere being positively charged, there's a difference in electrical potential between the two. Electrically charged streams from the Sun, called solar winds, interact with the rotating upper atmosphere like the brushes of an electrical generator. The resulting structure is what is called a magnetosphere, which is, in fact, a type of electrical generator; and the lower atmosphere, which forms a "cavity" between the Earth and the ionosphere, acts like a storage battery for the electrical potential that is built up. When conditions are right, we can see this process as the *aurora borealis* (in the Arctic) or *aurora australis* (in the Antarctic).

In the 1950s, German geophysicist Dr. W. O. Schumann suggested that this phenomenon might mean that electromagnetic signals circulate at extremely low frequencies in the gap between the Earth and the ionosphere. These signals came to be called "Schumann's Resonances" (SR). The frequencies of these SR signals increase or decrease with ionospheric conditions, which change daily, seasonally, with the lunar cycle, and with variations in solar activity, which, in turn, varies with the eleven-year sunspot cycle. So long as the properties of Earth's electromagnetic cavity remain about the same, these frequencies remain the same. They seem to be related only to electrical activity in the atmosphere, particularly during times of intense lightning activity. There's no evidence suggesting that they're caused by terrestrial factors like Earth's tectonic plate movements or even shifts in the Earth's core, even though those features do produce magnetic fields.

Like waves on a stringed musical instrument or on the ocean, SR must be potentiated or "excited" to be observed. They've been observed, by experiment, as occurring at several harmonic frequencies. Not too surprisingly, since we evolved as part of this terrestrial electrical system, these frequencies are the same cycles as typical theta (sleep) and beta (waking state) brain-wave rhythms documented on EEGs, and the blank range between the first two levels is a very reasonable match with the alpha (dreaming and light meditation) rhythm. The planet, it seems, exhibits the same states of consciousness as we do!

In their exploration of these ideas, Richard and Iona Miller suggest that

> Schumann's resonance forms a natural feedback loop with the human mind/body. The human brain and body developed in the biosphere, the [electromagnetic] environment conditioned by this cyclic pulse. Conversely, this pulse acts as a "driver" of our brains and can also potentially carry information. Functional processes may be altered and new patterns of behaviour facilitated through the brain's web of inhibitory and excitatory feedback networks. (Miller and Miller 2004)

They also suggest that, because oscillating patterns tend to set up resonance with other oscillating patterns, changes in Schumann's Resonances may lead to changes in the pattern of oscillation in our individual electromagnetic fields, and, conversely, the oscillation pattern of any individual may affect the patterns of those around that person and the larger field, as well.

Morphic Resonance

Rupert Sheldrake is an evolutionary biologist who sought to understand how it is that similar mutations in plants and animals have occurred across the planet at very nearly the same time without direct interaction. In his groundbreaking book, *A New Science of Life* (1981), Sheldrake offered a number of related examples and proposed a "Theory of Morphic Resonance" to explain them. Sheldrake hypothesized that the occurrence of an event anywhere increased the likelihood of the same event happening everywhere, all at once. He called the mechanism by which this might occur "resonating morphogenetic fields" (ibid.).

Such fields, he says, are not physical in the sense of being measurable by the usual electromagnetic devices, but they are more like resonating patterns of information encompassing the planet, which, when a life-form resonates with it, generates a new internal and external form for that life.

> ... morphogenetic fields differ radically from electromagnetic fields in that the latter depend on the *actual* state of the system—on the distribution and movement of charged particles—whereas morphogenetic fields correspond to the *potential* state of a developing system and are already present before it takes up its final form. (ibid., 77)

An example from human experience would be the process by which a secret scientific discovery is often repeated almost immediately elsewhere, long before anyone outside of the original laboratory knows about the first discovery.

One of Sheldrake's examples suggesting Morphic Resonance was with rats, many years before he proposed his theory. Generations of rats were trained to do a new task at Harvard, in Massachusetts. Some time later, a different group of rats were trained to do the same task in Edinburgh. The Edinburgh group learned the task far more quickly—some without even being trained (ibid., 189–90).

Since those early years, there have been hundreds of experiments testing the idea, with remarkable results. Sheldrake has since focused on the ability of pets to discern when their family members are coming home—even before the people are within sight or sound and are off any usual schedule (Sheldrake, McKenna, and Abraham 1998).

An intriguing aspect of this theory is its similarity to the model of human consciousness suggested by Carl Jung. In Jung's model, individual consciousness is seen as an open-ended field within a larger field, the collective consciousness. As presented by Markley and Harman in their seminal work, *Changing Images of Man* (1975,

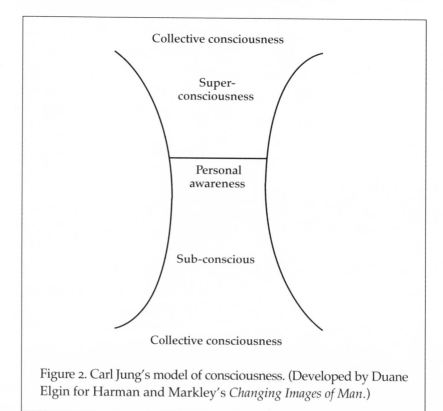

Figure 2. Carl Jung's model of consciousness. (Developed by Duane Elgin for Harman and Markley's *Changing Images of Man.*)

1984), the collective field is divided into the collective subconscious, associated with the darker emotions, fear, and attachment to matter, and the collective superconscious, associated with ideals. Jung's archetypes (ideas and forms that are present in dreams and stories across cultures) are located in this collective consciousness, accessible to and affecting the individual consciousness as the individual is ready to experience them—or, using Sheldrake's term, resonates with them.

Both the Morphic Resonance and the collective consciousness theories were developed apart from Schumann's work with atmospheric resonance, but both of them support and extend it. If, as the Millers have suggested, the electromagnetic oscillation pattern within the atmospheric cavity can carry information (which we know is true because that is exactly how radio works), then both archetypal structures and new insights or mutations could well be encoded in the resonant pattern of Earth's electromagnetic field. They would therefore be instantaneously available to any resonating energy pattern anywhere on the planet, just as a radio, tuned to the right frequency, can receive information from anywhere on the planet, almost as it is transmitted.

Biophysics

ONE OF THE MORE EXCITING DEVELOPMENTS in the world of science is the integration of the theory and practice of physics with the study of biological systems. As physicists look at cells and tissues, they see things that biologists could not—offering new understandings in the process.

Semiconductors

Once we accept the possibility of electromagnetic energy as a significant aspect of the mind-body system, whole new possibilities emerge and we start to see relationships that have not been clear before.

As biologists have studied the mechanism by which materials and information are passed through the outer "wall" or membrane of a cell, they have found two layers of permeable protein molecules with an impermeable layer of fat molecules between them ("like a butter sandwich"). Through this, only the matter or information whose electrical charge pattern conforms to that of certain molecular gateways, called receptors, penetrates into the interior of the cell. According to Bruce Lipton (2005), this "semi-conducting" nature of the cell wall is part of how the cell maintains its identity in a constantly changing environment.

Maret has developed this vision further, reminding us that

> ... medical schools and healers are not taught that the largest organ of the body is the connective tissue matrix. In the past this matrix was often simply seen as the stuff that glues the important organ systems of the body together. We are now realizing that it is here that the mysteries of life can be most fully explored.... (in Oschman 2000, ix)

The wave-form of our bodies is energy, but, if we really think about it, the matter-form of our bodies is mostly fluid. Even the bones, when studied in the body, are soft and resilient—unlike the hard and dry skeletons that we are shown in museums and laboratories. Children's bodies are typically 97 percent water, decreasing over the years to about 75 percent in elderly bodies. The connective tissue of the manifest body is mostly liquid and takes the form of long, thin molecules that are known as "liquid crystals." These liquid crystals transmit and receive signals in the body just as they do on a cell phone, laptop, or flat screen TV. Though they are a very different system from the nerve system, they nonetheless participate in the transfer of energy and information throughout the manifest body—in ways that correspond to the *nadis* and acupressure nodes of the Eastern model of the mind-body.

Maret challenges us further, to shift our thinking about the body from a focus on the individual parts to the functioning whole.

> An inspired vision of this emerging medicine emphasizes the importance of the living tissue matrix with its unique properties of semiconducting proteins, liquid crystalline holographic structure, vicinal water domains ... and almost instantaneous, faster than nerve conduction, information transfer.... Here cells are seen as fractals embedded in a holographic energetic matrix where everything is interconnected and capable of influencing every other part of the matrix. Information can be communicated through ... photons of ultraviolet and visible light, phonons of sound, multiple resonant cellular vibrations, charge density waves and quantum potentials. The body becomes visible as a living, energetic whole even though composed of specialized organ systems and cellular aggregates. Ultimately, a picture of an electromagnetically unified matrix containing a self-organizing blueprint with innumerable feedback loops begins to emerge. (in Oschman 2000, ix)

Maret's vision helps us to shift from a view of the mind-body limited by the solid structures we can measure to a tightly interconnected structure of electromagnetic processes, based in an energy-form with many of the qualities of light.

Living Systems

Through the last decades of the twentieth century, as mathematicians, ecologists, and systems thinkers explored the behavior and evolution of complex systems, the set of ideas called Living Systems Theory emerged. It integrates these disciplines into a body of principles that apply to all living organisms, including human social organizations.

The first principle of all systems theory is that everything is interconnected and we can never do just one thing. In living systems, this is demonstrated by the fact that one cannot affect a part of a body without affecting other parts of the body: cannot, for example, injure a foot without affecting the posture, which may lead to spinal injury at the worst—or simply aching shoulders. Nor can we introduce a chemical—say, an antibiotic to kill an infectious bacterium—without affecting other aspects of the system: the antibiotic will also kill the "good" bacteria that live in the intestines and help us digest foods.

A second principle of Living Systems Theory is that even when things look chaotic, there is order; and vice versa: the most orderly processes include a degree of chaos. The underlying order of a forest or a pond may not be evident until a part is injured or removed—then, the resulting shifts and changes demonstrate the order that was present before. The orderly process of development in the fetus or from infant to adult seems, at times, to be chaotic, but in hindsight we can see how each individual event contributes to, and often contains the pattern of, the whole process.

A third principle is that of nonlinearity. Living systems grow exponentially, following an "S" shaped curve on a graph, and are sustainable within a range of limits between which they oscillate over time. As the Episcopalian-priest-turned-Buddhist-philosopher Alan Watts used to say, "Nature is wiggly." Continuous growth is as unhealthy in living systems as continuous decline—and will almost invariably lead to catastrophic results.

A fourth principle is that of "dissipative structures." The term was coined by Nobel laureate Ilya Prigogine (1984) to describe the process by which systems and most structures exist only as long as energy continues to flow into them and through them. Clearly, this is a primary characteristic of living systems. Prigogine also suggests that when the flow that sustains the structure changes, the structure may collapse or dissipate, or it may respond by restructuring in a way that can be sustained with the new level of energy flow. Many researchers have used this principle to explain evolutionary processes by which living systems increase in complexity, rather than decay due to entropy as most physical structures must.

This increase in complexity happens through the fifth principle that defines living systems: self-organization through feedback. All living systems develop from apparently inert "seeds of potentiality" into more or less complex dynamic bodies. They take in matter and energy from the environment, combine it in unique patterns, and form new structures with new capabilities through a series of developmental stages. Through these processes, information about the environment, the substances taken in, the current state of the system, and the outputs is passed around within the system and between it and its environment. This information is "fed back" to the processors in the system to adjust their activity.

A living systems perspective, therefore, says that the human mind-body is an interconnected whole within a larger interconnected whole, within which we can "never do just one thing." The mind-body develops in an orderly process that sometimes feels chaotic and is "wiggly" rather than linear. It is maintained by a continuous flow of energy and, if that flow shifts, the mind-body must restructure to function at the new level or it will dissipate or collapse.

An Integrated Model

THERE ARE, PERHAPS, thousands of models of the human mind-body system. Every cultural and philosophical tradition on the planet must develop one in order to make sense of human experience. We recognize this and are humbled by the fact. We do not wish to set our ideas above any others; we wish simply to discover a way of thinking about the body that allows for, and perhaps explains, the many and varied therapeutic experiences that we've practiced and observed.

Thus far, we have identified several elements of an explanatory model for the physical structure of the human mind-body system:

1. Mind and body are physically, chemically, and energetically inseparable.

2. That which we call the body is not a solid, fixed object but at its most basic level is a dynamic set of interacting fields of energy, oscillating in a unique resonant pattern.

3. The energy fields of which we are composed and those that we generate range in frequency across the electromagnetic spectrum, including both perceivable and imperceptible levels of light and other forms of energy.

4. These fields interact in such a way that cells, tissue, and organs develop and are maintained as the manifest mind-body.

5. The manifest mind-body is sustained by an oscillating flow of energy through the energy fields and cellular structures that constitute it.

6. The energy fields and the manifest mind-body they sustain are part of, affect, and are affected by a larger set of electromagnetic energy fields, surrounding the planet and pervading the solar system, through which flows energy that sustains the mind-body.

Thus far, the model of the mind-body we are developing is structured within—and sustained by—a set of interacting energy fields, which are, in turn, interacting with larger energy fields that sustain them. As we continue,

7. Flows and interactions in the energy fields of the mind-body can be blocked, pulled out of balance, or enhanced, which directly affects function in the manifest mind-body.

8. Blocks and imbalances may emerge through interactions with other, nonresonating energy fields, or through patterns of thought and feeling.

9. The mind-body's interacting energy fields can be restored to balance or enhanced through various forms of meditation,

including visualization; frequent visualization of these energy fields as light brings the matter-energy system into balance and enhances the capabilities and well-being of the manifest mind-body.

In our model, then, disruption of flows in the energy body leads to disturbances in the manifest body. These disruptions may be the result of interference from other energy fields but are more often a function of our own thoughts and feelings, upsetting the balances. Not only can we disrupt the flows, we can also enhance the flows—thereby enhancing function—by shifting our inner focus so we can perceive the energy fields of the body as kinds of light.

However, beyond the energy body and the manifest, physical body that it sustains, we've seen that who we are functions through other dimensions, as well. Our experience as a species has made it clear that we are not isolated individuals, and we are capable of experiencing and expressing our nature throughout space-time, instantly. Aspects of ourselves function outside of three-dimensional reality, in the subtle bodies and what the Buddhists call the *trikaya*:

10. One other-dimensional aspect is the body of awareness, the *Nirmanakaya*, causal body, *Atman*, Oversoul, or Higher Self.

11. Another aspect is the body of radiant communication, the *Sambhogakaya*, etheric/celestial body, or Christ Consciousness.

12. Then there is the universal field potential unique to each being and interacting with all other beings, the *Dharmakaya, Brahman, rigpa*, or Holy Spirit.

This model, then, defines the individual mind-body that we call ourself as the unique pattern of interactions among these aspects of one multifold body, with its heart-centered resonating rhythms, along with the pattern of interaction with the larger system of energy fields and bodies that surround it.

To place this model in an experiential context, consider the following possibility (a true story):

As you move through the day, you realize that things aren't quite working. You feel a little out of sorts, you are stopped at every stoplight, and you spill your beverage when you reach for something else across the table. About that point, someone walks up to you and tells you all the things you did wrong on a recent task. It feels awful, but you go ahead, doing your job and trying not to think about it. You become aware of a vague ache around the eyes.

Lunch time comes and you've agreed to meet a friend. You head for the door and drop your keys on the way to the car. You fumble your way into the car and drop something else as you reach to put the keys into the ignition.

About that time you stop. You wake up. You realize that this pattern is not working and more, that it's not who you are or how you intend to live your life.

With that realization, you close your eyes and take a deep breath, relaxing into your body, there, in the driver's seat of your car. You take another deep breath, letting all the tension that's been accumulating in your shoulders, neck, and facial muscles release and dissolve. You sit there, for a moment, simply breathing. This feels better.

Then you open your eyes and look up. Above the cars, above the buildings, is the great dome of the sky. You see the beauty in the sky, the patterns of light, and you appreciate them. As you do so, you feel a deeper release in your body. An even more comfortable sensation.

Suddenly, a bird flies toward you, landing almost on the car you're sitting in. It cocks its head and looks directly at you, as if to say "I know who you are; we're connected!" It stays for several moments, looking at you. You see the beautiful markings on its wings and face, the delicate pattern of its feathers, and you are awed by the beauty and complexity they display. Then the bird chirps a couple of times and, in a delightful sweep, takes off. You smile. What an amazing event! What an amazing thing life is!

You look at your clock. Incredibly, only one minute has passed since you stumbled your way into the car, but you feel like a new person.

Eyes open, aware of all the sights and sounds around you, you take another deep breath, down into your belly. This time you *feel*, you *see* with your inner eye, a swirl of light moving through your body with your breath. And as you do so you become aware that there's an open space around your heart. A new kind of light seems to be moving through you. You close your eyes, following that light through your heart *chakra*. As you do so, a "thrill of cool fire" moves through your body—what some people call "God bumps." You smile in appreciation and continue to focus on that opening at your heart.

There, in that opening, you feel the infinite potential of all that is, there for you, waiting to be realized. Sitting there, filled with energy, you allow that potential to come forth through you, resting your sense of self in it, feeling it emanate out from you in all directions, carrying your appreciations and intentions with it.

So you remember the criticism you received earlier and, in this state of Grace, you release it, knowing that it is not the truth about you or your work. You release it and let it go, claiming the higher truth, the deeper knowing, of this state of being you're experiencing now. Sitting there, at this moment, you realize, fully, that in Truth, all is well. And as that thought appears, it spins outward with the energy of potential emerging from your heart *chakra*. As you follow it with your inner vision, you feel that *chakra* shut down. The "wormhole"[16] has closed and you no longer experience yourself as the other-

---

16. "Wormhole" is the term used in science fiction for a place through which one can move into other dimensions.

dimensional body, the *Dharmakaya*, but simply you, feeling well and happy and about to be late for lunch.

You look at the clock again—incredibly, only another minute has passed! You'll be on time, after all! Truly all is well!

As you buckle up and turn on the ignition, the cell phone rings. Someone on the other side of the continent just got the word that, because of that task you were just criticized about, you've been invited to a significant event—something that would mean a lot to you and others—and all expenses will be paid. Your smile turns into a grin. As you cruise down the road, watching the green lights go by, you can't help but think, What a wonderful world this is!

Clearly, this is a radical departure from the way most of us have been taught to think about our bodies and how they work. Equally clearly, Western scientific medicine as it has evolved cannot provide effective methods for working with this new model. This is no longer Era I. We have entered Era II medicine and are preparing the way for Era III. Fortunately, methods are available that can work—and new ones are being created, all the time.

References

Bentov, Itzhak. *Stalking the Wild Pendulum*. Rochester, VT: Destiny Books, 1977.

Brennan, Barbara. *Hands of Light*. New York: Bantam, 1990.

Capra, Fritjof. *The Tao of Physics*. New York: Bantam, 1984.

Castaneda, Carlos. *The Active Side of Infinity*. Toronto: HarperCollins Canada, 1998.

Chang, G. C. C. *Six Yogas of Naropa*. Ithaca, NY: Snow Lion, 1963.

Cousins, Norman. *Anatomy of an Illness from a Patient's Perspective*. New York: Norton, 1979.

Dudjom Rinpoche. *Counsels from My Heart*. Boston: Shambhala, 2001.

Freemantle, Francesca. *Luminous Emptiness*. Boston: Shambhala, 2001.

Frölich, Herbert. "Coherent Excitations in Active Biological Systems." In Felix Gutmann and Hendrik Keyzer. *Modern Bioelectrochemistry*. New York: Plenum, 1986.

Gerber, Richard. *Vibrational Medicine*. Santa Fe, NM: Bear, 1988.

Goswami, Amit. *The Self-Aware Universe*. New York: Tarcher/Putnam, 1993.

Govindan, Marshall. *Babaji and the 18 Siddha Kriya Yoga Tradition*. Montreal: Kriya Yoga Publications, 1991.

Greiner, Walter, and Aurel Sandulescu. "New Radioactivities." *Scientific American* (March 1990).

Hudson, David. "Alchemy: Portland Presentation." Video. 1998.

Kaptchuk, Ted J. *The Web That Has No Weaver*. New York: Congdon & Weed, 1983.

Khalsa, Dharma S. *Meditation as Medicine*. New York: Simon & Schuster, 2001.

Lipton, Bruce. *The Biology of Belief*. Santa Rosa, CA: Elite Press, 2005.

Lo, Pei-Chen, Ming-Liang Huang, and Kang-Ming Chang. "EEG Alpha Blocking Correlated with Perception of Inner Light During Zen Meditation." *American Journal of Chinese Medicine* 31, no. 4 (2003): 629–42.

Markley, Oliver W., and Willis Harman. *Changing Images of Man*. Menlo Park, CA: Stanford Research Institute, 1975; New York: Pergamon, 1984.

Mead, G. R. S. *The Doctrine of the Subtle Body in Western Tradition*. Wheaton, IL: Quest, 1919, 1967.

Miller, Iona, and Richard Miller. "Biophysics/Mindbody." nexusmagazine.com, 2004.

Miller, Ruth L. *150 Years of Healing*. Portland, OR: Abib, 2000.

Myss, Caroline. *The Anatomy of the Spirit*. New York: Harmony Books, 1994.

Ornstein, Robert. *Psychology of Consciousness*. New York: Viking, 1972.

Oschman, James. *Energy Medicine: The Scientific Basis.* London: Churchill, 2000.

Physical Review Letters 62, no. 10 (March 6, 1989).

Popp, Fritz-Albert. "Physical Aspects of Biophotons." *Experientia* 44 (1988): 576–85.

Prigogine, Ilya. *Order Out of Chaos.* Toronto: Bantam, 1984.

Puthoff, Harold E. "Everything for Nothing." *New Scientist* (July 28, 1990).

Rama, Swami, Rudolph Ballentine, and Alan Hymes. *Science of Breath.* Honesdale, PA: Himalayan International Institute, 1979.

Sheldrake, Rupert. *A New Science of Life.* Los Angeles: Tarcher, 1981.

Sheldrake, Rupert, Terence McKenna, and Ralph Abraham. *The Evolutionary Mind.* Santa Cruz, CA: Trialogue Press, 1998.

Sogyal Rinpoche. *The Tibetan Book of Living and Dying.* New York: HarperCollins, 1994.

Norbu, Thinley. *The Small Golden Key.* New York: Jewel, 1985.

Thondup, Tulku. *The Practice of Dzogchen: Writings of Longchen Rabjam.* Ithaca, NY: Snow Lion, 1989.

Winner, Anne Kennedy. *The Basic Ideas of Occult Wisdom.* Wheaton, IL: Quest, 1970.

Zohar, Danah. *The Quantum Self: Human Nature and Consciousness Defined by the New Physics.* New York: William Morrow, 1990.

CHAPTER 6

A New Model
of the Healing Process

AS LONG AS THE BODY WAS SEEN AS A SET of interchangeable mechanical parts, held together by a complex biochemical processor, healing was a function of replacing worn-out or broken parts or providing the appropriate chemical. However, as soon as we acknowledge that thought, emotions, and mental imagery play a role in the healing process—on the part of both the patient and the care provider—then a very different description of the healing process becomes necessary. A new model of the human mind-body suggests a new model for the healing process, as well.

As we understand more about the dynamics of the mind-body system, we can see that many of the assumptions and expectations of Western "scientific medicine" may create more problems than they solve. A new model of healing works holistically, seeing the mind-body system as a set of interacting elements sustained by constant energy flows. Healers working from such a model would not suddenly shift those energy flows, recognizing that too great a fluctuation could result in the collapse of the system. Nor would they expect fixed or constant behaviors, but would recognize a range of possible states as "normal" and would not encourage static states or continuous movement in any particular direction. Recognizing the complex set of interactions making up the person before them, they would tend to seek a dynamic equilibrium rather than an ideal state, and they would teach their patients how to achieve and maintain that equilibrium on their own, in relationship with friends and family.

As we understand more clearly the structure of the mind-body, we begin to shift our assumptions and expectations about the nature of its condition. Because the condition of the manifest body is a function of what is happening in the energy fields and in their inter-action with the manifest body through the many energy channels, seeing the energy body as an effective model of human function becomes a diagnostic tool. Numerous "medical intuitives," such as Jane Katra, coauthor of *Miracles of Mind* (Targ and Katra 1999), Judith Orloff, and Caroline Myss, as presented in *The Anatomy of the Spirit* (1994), have demonstrated its utility in countless situations, and physicians like Norman Shealy and Larry Dossey have learned to rely on such understandings:

> Anyone who is aware of the recent trends in medicine will realize that modern physicians—like the physicists before them—have begun to deal with finer and finer forms of energy both in the diagnosis and treatment of human illness. (Dossey, endorsement of Richard Gerber's *Vibrational Medicine* 1988)

As we understand more fully the interactive relationship between any individual and the living systems in which that indi-vidual acts, we begin to integrate more people into our treatment protocols, and we pay more attention to the interpersonal and transpersonal context in which the individual is operating.

Transpersonal Medicine

IN HIS COMPREHENSIVE STUDY, *Transpersonal Medicine*, Frank Lawlis, a medical doctor trained in traditional, allopathic institutions, has done a remarkable job of identifying the major concerns and contributions in the field, starting with the proposition that,

At its root, transpersonal medicine recognizes that the power of love, compassion, community, and intention are as important to healing as any of our pills and medicines, and possibly more powerful ... (Lawlis 1996, xvi)

Lawlis became interested in transpersonal approaches as he worked to help patients control pain. He states that transpersonal medicine is

... based on people's experience of transcending their usual identification with their limited biological, historical, cultural, and personal selves and, at the most profound levels of experience possible, recognizing or even being "something" of vast intelligence and compassion that encompasses the entire universe.... the transpersonal, which experientially impresses us with our fundamental unity with each other and all life ... (ibid., 5)

As Lawlis continued his research, he discovered the work of Jeanne Achterberg, who has pointed out the importance of ritual in healing processes across cultures (1985). In *Transpersonal Medicine,* he quotes her as saying that ritual is "the universal foundation for all transpersonal medicine" (Lawlis 1996, 6). Regular, repeated practice is one of the definitions of the word *ritual,* and part of the process that gives the necessary depth of meaning to the symbols.

Observing the wide range of responses to pain medication among his patients—a range that seemed to have far less to do with the patient's bodyweight and health than with the patient's state of mind and community—Dr. Frank Lawlis started to experiment with different approaches. Visualization, Progressive Relaxation, and listening were among the techniques he found effective, with consistently higher results in cases where groups worked together to support individuals.

This is not surprising, because all the guidelines for effective imagery start with the same instructions: relax the body and still the mind, focusing on the emerging image and letting awareness of external events slip away. Clearly, these guidelines elicit Benson's Relaxation Response, which has been found to be so effective in encouraging a sense of well-being. The additional effects of the inner "experience" provided by the imagery session augment the overall effectiveness of this technique.

Recent studies, such as those supported by the Institute of Noetic Sciences, have gone even further than Lawlis' experience, demonstrating that not only the thoughts and beliefs of the patient, but those of the doctor and other caregivers, affect the patient's recovery. Several hundred studies focusing on the effects of prayer—by doctors and other staff, by friends and family, and by strangers—observing several thousand patients under a variety of experimental designs, have established that the kind of intense positive regard with an intention of well-being for the patient that we call prayer results in significant improvements in responses to medical procedures, speeds recovery from such procedures, and reduces the number and severity of side effects associated with the procedures and with hospital care (Dossey 1999; Schlitz et al. 2005; Murphy 1992).

Other studies, using placebos, have established a direct correlation between the caregiver's beliefs and the patient's response to the supposed treatment being offered. Among the most famous of these was the realization by a cardiologist that a common surgery for a specific heart problem did not, in fact, affect that problem, in spite of the consistently high rate of recovery for those who had gone through it (Cousins 1981).

The implications of these ideas for the healing process are substantial. First, it becomes necessary to recognize that the beliefs and attitudes of the care provider will affect the healing process of the patient. Beyond that, it becomes clear that whatever ideas or states are active in the collective consciousness will affect the individual—and vice versa—so the healer needs to be aware of the larger picture while addressing the local issue.

The Power of Intention

INTENTION TO HEAL OTHERS is a gift of human spirit inherent in the mind-body system. In health or in illness, at any time, the energy of healing intention that one radiates into oneself or out to another person, or to several other people, really helps relieve sickness and suffering. Clinical trials have proved that healing intention can be instantaneously used and directed by average people, that it is not the special gift of a few "healers." Indeed, it seems to be a gift that most or all people have and can use, which is why so many people have benefited from energy healing practices, in spite of the relatively little-known research to support its value.

What is the energy of intention? It's something more readily experienced than explained. The energy of intention is akin to the energy of prayer, which is described as nonphysical (Dossey 1993). It is experienced not as something traveling through air or space, through which it might deteriorate, but as reaching its destination full-force, and instantly, in the unified field of life.

This characteristic of healing intention is in accordance with our model of the body, because what shifts is the practitioner's own energy field, which instantaneously affects all the energy fields resonating with it across the planet. Such is our unlimited, universal nature

The intention to heal, as *Reiki* and other energy practitioners learn, begins a healing process for the practitioner as well as the receiver. Then the focus on a particular person establishes the resonant connection for the healing/healed field of the practitioner to interact with the corresponding field of the receiver—and any other similar resonances along the way. Such is the nature of resonant vibration.

Another property of the energy of healing intention is that it is integral to the light nature of the body, called the *Sambhogakaya* by

Buddhists, and seems to work outside of normal time and space. This suggests that the source of the power of healing intention is both our *Dharmakaya*, or infinite nature, and the *Nirmanakaya*, our causal body.

Energy Healing Methods

GIVEN A MODEL of the human body that is based on energy, the inclusion of energy healing methods in our model of healing seems imperative. Typically, such methods as acupuncture, acupressure, reflexology, and some forms of chiropractic require extensive training for the practitioner in both diagnostic and therapeutic methods. Other energy methods, including Therapeutic or Healing Touch, *Reiki*, laying on of hands, and use of crystals, are more easily learned and applied. The practitioner is trained to both diagnose the condition by "reading" the energy and treat the condition by letting energy flow through them into the patient. A practitioner may also self-administer these forms of healing. In fact, some trainers encourage students to do so as a way to practice the method. Training in these methods is relatively inexpensive and available, making them far more accessible than many healing modalities.

Most energy healing methods assume our model's principle that dysfunction in the manifest body is first a dysfunction in the energy body. Practitioners are trained to "read" the patterns in the field of energy around the body to identify potential problem areas and then they allow what we've called *chi* or *prana*, the universal life force, to flow through their own central energy channel and out through their hands to the affected energy center or physical body part.

For *Reiki* practitioners (*Reiki* meaning "universal life energy"), it's possible to obtain additional training to learn how to "send" life force across space and time—for both diagnosis and healing. This "second-degree" training also provides techniques for discovering blocks in the energy channels and dissolving them. In terms of our model, of course, the only thing being "sent" is the intention—a shift in one's own energy field that resonates with the energy of the other and assists a shift there toward greater harmony and balance.

The use of needles or crystals in these methods enhances the energy shift by either pinpointing it to specific energy channels (in the case of acupuncture) or (in the case of crystals) tuning the energy flowing from the practitioner to a specific frequency to better meet the needs of the patient.

In all energy methods, the practitioner's role is to permit the energy to flow through them (or their needles or crystals) into the patient's energy system. In terms of our model, the practitioner is using intention and imagery to restore harmony in the shared energy body of the practitioner and patient, thus facilitating a restoration of health in the manifest, physical body.

The Role of Meditation

IN ALL OF THE RESEARCH cited in Chapter Three of this book, one thing is perfectly clear: the practice of meditation significantly enhances the well-being of the practitioner, regardless of age or state of health when begun, and without the negative side effects of invasive, Era I techniques. In terms of the model we have developed here, we can say that the practice of meditation assists the manifest body directly through rest and relaxation, and enhances the function of the energy body by allowing the energy fields and channels to be re-balanced and replenished.

As we consider the use of meditation as a form of therapy appropriate to an Era II or Era III model of medicine, we realize that all healing depends on the kinds of results that are achieved through the practice. Then it is a matter of discovering which of the different forms of meditation are most appropriate for which kinds of conditions.

Imagery

Although not usually considered a form of meditation in the classic Buddhist sense, many of the same characteristics apply. Imagery requires stopping what one is doing and focusing on an internal process, thus resting the body and ending normal thought processes. Imagery also can be experienced as a process of alignment, harmonizing different aspects of the mind-body, in ways that are very much like what researchers have found that certain dream states provide.

As Lawlis discovered in his pain clinics, imagining being healthy or an experience of becoming healthy can be very effective in reducing the discomfort of symptoms, and often the symptoms themselves. Imagery, in all its forms, can be used to shift a patient's focus from his or her distress, to create an alternative understanding of the situation and, through repetition, to replace old patterns of worry or fixation on the past with a new pattern of thought and feeling. This last form, commonly called "positive imagery," has been proved effective in athletics and the workplace, as well as in therapeutic settings.

Imagery is most typically used in association with chronic conditions and terminal illness. However, increasing experience with the technique proves it to be useful for reducing swelling and inflammation (decreasing pain and sinus problems), shifting blood flow from the brain to the extremities (reducing or eliminating headaches), and removing excess inches from the body (most effectively as part of a plan of diet and exercise).

Progressive Relaxation Therapies

Because of Edmund Jacobson's remarkable work demonstrating the effectiveness of progressive neuromuscular release, and through Kabat-Zinn's application of that method in his work with mindfulness meditation, we have a body of evidence and protocol for its use, and a clear understanding of the conditions that are most amenable to treatment with this method.

Indications for treatment by Progressive Relaxation include:

- acute neuromuscular hypertension
- chronic neuromuscular hypertension
- states of fatigue and exhaustion
- states of debility (convalescence from infectious and exhaustive diseases of various types)
- chronic pulmonary tuberculosis
- organic and functional heart disorders
- vascular hypertension
- preoperative and postoperative conditions
- toxic goiter
- disturbances of sleep
- alimentary spasm, including mucous colitis, colonic spasm, cardiospasm, and esophagospasm
- peptic ulcer
- preventive medicine

Vase Breathing: Awareness-Based Energy Breathing

For centuries, breathing energy into the navel area has been known to be a great method for developing and maintaining optimal human function.

Vase Breathing is energy breathing in energy body, which is doubly transformative. There is a totally different sense of what breathes and what is breathed. In addition, the profound developmental shift from mind to awareness is identical with that found in mindfulness (*Vipashyana*) meditation. Dr. Dean Ornish has included a form of energy breathing in his plan for heart patients.

It is a central concern of this book, given the great medical potential of Vase Breathing, to encourage research to ascertain its benefits. Mindfulness meditation has been substantially researched, with great interest in the medical value of its benefits. Vase Breathing has the same central psychological method as mindfulness meditation but may have even more profound biological and psychological benefits because of its impact on deeper dimensions of body and breathing. We hope that research will soon support the application of Vase Breathing in medicine at least as much as it supports the application of mindfulness meditation.

Based on experience and known functionality, medical indications for the use of Vase Breathing include:

- general medicine
- cancer care
- coronary care
- HIV / AIDS care
- high-anxiety care
- depression care
- immune enhancement
- pain management
- complications from medication and surgery
- near-death care
- childbirth medicine

Transformative Compassionate Breathing

In Compassionate Breathing, breath becomes very powerful. Simply going with the natural flow of the breath, one breathes in, taking into the energy body the energy of the apparent sickness and suffering of any living person—oneself or anyone else. The energy breathed in dissolves into light in the energy body, and then healing energy is breathed out into whomever one intends to heal, wherever they are. The nonlocal nature of our mind-body means that we can merge our intention with another and it is felt by the person we focus on, along with all others with similar patterns of energy.

A powerful illustration of this method occurred in Tibet, in the eleventh century. Leprosy was common, and ordinary doctors didn't know how to cure it. Perhaps it could be compared to AIDS today. A lama named Geshe Chekhawa taught Compassionate Breathing, called *Tong Len*, in Tibet, to a group of lepers. "Many of the lepers who did *Tong Len* practice were cured. The news of this spread fast, and many other lepers flocked to his house" (Sogyal 1994, 194).

Let's apply this in today's terms. A person suffering with leprosy, or AIDS, goes to a lama, a spiritual teacher, pleading for help. The teacher says to that person that there is a method that might be able to cure them. The suffering person would have to practice the method by himself, or herself, and practice it intensively. The essence of it is that they would have to be willing to drop their suffering, to forget about it, and compassionately open their heart to another suffering person, someone suffering the same disease. They practice healing others and themselves, using their inherent healing ability, rather than focusing on their own suffering. The more completely the practice is done, they're told, the more likely it will be to bring healing to the person who does the practice.

Describing compassion or *Bodhicitta* (*bodhi* meaning "enlightened essence" and *citta* meaning "heart"), Shantideva writes:

It is the supreme elixir
that overcomes the sovereignty of death.
It is the inexhaustible treasure
that eliminates poverty in the world.
It is the supreme medicine
that quells the world's disease. (ibid., 201)

When people drop their suffering self-nature and turn attention to another aspect of their mind-body, they shift into the innate, unconditioned functioning of the *Nirmanakaya* or causal body. It's possible to quickly dissolve the obstructions resulting from one's conditioned functioning because one is inherently free of that conditioning. One can turn directly to one's life force and enter the great potential of *Dharmakaya,* unlimited power, removing all obstructions to one's own health. Compassionate Breathing for oneself and others doesn't waste a breath.

As a result, Compassionate Breathing is a form of meditation that may be applied to any condition involving prolonged distress or suffering. It has been effectively used for the labor of childbirth, as well as such conditions as AIDS, rheumatoid arthritis, osteoarthritis, and cancers.

Audio-Guidance

People who are semi-comatose, such as those suffering from Alzheimer's disease, those who are in deep coma, and those who are near death require health care methods that cover a vast range of concerns. This is an area of health care for which the methods of Era I medicine are considered inappropriate by many people, among them health care professionals and a large portion of the general public. We see controversial and expensive medical interventions used aggressively, often without improving the quality of life of the patients—who, all too often, have been subjected to such treatment without informed consent. These are health care fields where new methods and approaches are crucially needed.

Toward the end of his life, Carl Jung reflected on

> ... certain astonishing observations in cases of profound [unconsciousness] after acute injuries to the brain and in severe cases of [brain] collapse. In both situations, total loss of consciousness can be accompanied by perceptions of the outside world and vivid dream experiences. Since the cerebral

cortex, the seat of consciousness, is not functioning at these times, there is as yet no explanation for such phenomena. They may be evidence for at least a subjective persistence of the capacity for consciousness—even in a state of apparent unconsciousness. (1961, 322)

Jung's "astonishing observation" concerning the indestructible and perhaps undisturbable foundation for mental activity, which we have called "inner awareness," may have been an anticipation of the turning to meditation methods in the West. Today, countless thousands of people in Western nations are discovering the nature of the inner awareness: timeless, immortal, and experientially free of disturbance and limitation.

In considering an approach to comatose, semi-comatose, and near-death states, it's useful to note that all three situations have one vital common factor: functioning in the outer world is no longer a matter of concern to that person. For each of these conditions, the ability to access inner awareness has become the important thing. Because there is diminished concern for the outer world, inner awareness is more accessible. Therefore, the approach with highest potential for effectiveness in all these conditions is one that addresses the need to access inner awareness: meditation.

The question becomes, however, how can one arrange for a demented or comatose patient to meditate? One promising solution is a pre-recorded guided meditation that can be played near the patient, regardless of location, activity, or condition. MediGrace, a nonprofit corporation directed by one of the authors, Robert Newman, produces such recordings, calling them "audio-guides." Health care providers who have used them have found them to be highly effective in reducing the severity of symptoms in their patients, reducing stress for caregivers, and providing the means for inner release. In some cases this may allow recovery.

Attitudinal Healing Methods

IN HIS REMARKABLE BOOK, *Teach Only Love* (1992), psychiatrist Gerald Jampolsky describes his movement from the limitations of his training into the infinite possibility of unconditional love and acceptance. Framed in the context of the teachings and principles of *A Course in Miracles*, Jampolsky's book outlines his transformative journey from diagnostics and treatment through loss of faith in healing to a new understanding of the nature of the therapeutic process and his own capacity to heal.

The outcome of the journey was the formation of the Center for Attitudinal Healing, presently located in Sausalito, California—which still functions, three decades after its founding.

What Jampolsky came to understand—and embodied in his Center—was that there is neither patient nor therapist, but two seekers together on a journey of healing. He accepted what many therapists know but do not acknowledge in their practice: that when the therapist is ready, the patient appears—exactly the perfect patient to help the therapist complete his or her own healing process. Beyond that, he realized that the really important function of the therapist operating in the traditional model is as Listener. It was not his expertise in pharmaceuticals, nor his demonstrated ability to apply various therapeutic models, that his patients needed. It was simply his ability to sit and focus and listen, without judgment, to what they needed to express.

So, Jampolsky made a decision. He decided to change his own attitude. He decided to let go of his persona as authoritative expert and all the judgments and assessments that went with that. He decided to focus, instead, on listening to, and loving (that is, accepting unconditionally, without attachment) his patients, and, in the process, he became a healer.

Not too surprisingly, this approach is very similar to the process of pastoral counseling that has recently begun to be taught to ministers, priests, and rabbis. It works—for both the counselor and the counselee.

In terms of the model presented here, what Jampolsky did was shift from Era I, invasive medicine to Era III, transpersonal medicine. He stopped operating as if the patient were a body with emotions and started seeing the whole, complex being—including the multidimensional bodies that are not always visible. He started to acknowledge that he could never do just one thing, and recognized that for either participant in the healing process to experience a greater degree of wholeness was for both of them to—and he let the patient guide the process, more often than not.

When we change our attitude, we do, in fact, change the pattern of energy that we are in the world, and the world responds accordingly.

The Healer

THE WESTERN ERA I MEDICAL TRADITION assumes that the patient is a passive receiver of healing modalities provided by a knowledgeable physician and his assistants. In Era I medicine it is the technique used or the medicine applied that makes the difference between illness and health. Though some physicians will go so far as to say that they are "helping the body to heal itself," recognizing the amazing, complex systems within the body for restoring well-being, most are convinced that it is the tools they use that do the work.

In the shamanic traditions, healing is a process that involves body, mind, spirit, and community. The patient is seen as an active participant in the healing process, along with friends and family. Individualized protocols are developed to assist the patient through the specific combination of actions and experiences that will undo the distress and restore well-being for all concerned. Often these include some forms of medicine, along with some psycho-emotional experiences and, often, spiritual counseling. The healer's role is that of facilitator.

The various energy healing methods fall somewhere in between these two models. The healer acts as a conduit of energy and a perceiver of specific blocks to energy flows, with the expectation that the patient's will and openness allow the energy to do its work in the body. It's understood that maintaining a healthy flow of energy to and through all parts of the body is essential for well-being and that the healer's role is to assist the patient in re-creating such a flow.

Mental healers operate on the assumption that the body is a record of the conscious and subconscious thoughts and feelings in the mind. They work to remove patterns of thought and feeling that cause distress in the body and to replace them with ways of thinking and feeling that restore well-being. The founders of the New Thought movement were adept at this mode of healing, both in direct contact and at a distance. Recognizing that the body tends toward health when its normal processes are not interfered with, they would find the specific set of words or thoughts that would undo the effects of the patient's old thought patterns and allow the body to resume its normal function.

In all of these methods, healers are approaching the distressed person not as a mechanical structure but as a complex energetic system that may be influenced by thought as well as action.

An Integrated Model of the Healing Process

A S WE CONSIDER EACH of these healing approaches in light of the model of the human body that we have offered, we can explain the role they play in bringing about a new, more fully functional state of being.

The basis of our model of the mind-body system is a set of interacting energy fields whose pattern of interaction leads to the manifestation of a material body, with its cells, tissue, and organs. Examining the healing methods described in this chapter, we can see that the energy associated with prayer, positive imagery, and listening with love has the effect of restoring a harmonious energy pattern where there has been dysfunction. The meditation practices of Progressive Relaxation and Vase Breathing permit the individual to rest in the harmony innate in the multidimensional body, thereby restoring that harmony and balance within the energy body and the physical body that it manifests.

Another element of our model is that dysfunction occurs first in the energy body, either through misaligned fields or through blocked energy channels. Clearly, the energy healing methods are useful for addressing these issues—either self-administered or provided by a trained practitioner. In addition, the meditation technique of Vase Breathing is specifically designed to restore harmony and balance to the fields and structures of the energy body.

A third, major element in our model is the transpersonal nature of the mind-body system. Being fully and continually in interaction with all other beings on the planet, we need healing methods that honor those connections and help us to utilize them effectively. The methods of prayer, distance *Reiki,* and Compassionate Breathing all honor the transpersonal nature of our being and give us means for shifting our attention from our own concerns to the concerns of others—and their healing—while simultaneously drawing into our energy body the necessary energy for healing ourselves.

Finally, our model states that, through our wave-form, otherdimensional bodies, human beings have the potential for operating not only everywhere on this planet at any instant, but everywhere in infinite dimensions. When the energy body is out of alignment, the flow of universal energy through these bodies into the mind-body system is impaired and the system may dissipate as a result.

Healing, in such cases, may take one of two directions. If the body has dissipated to the point where the consciousness is separating from it, healing comes in the form of audio-guidance into the next stage of life—called by many, death. If the choice is to remain connected, then the use of imagery and prayer to restore the flow is essential, supported by energy healing methods and the attitudinal healing of unconditional love. These methods have the capacity to restore function when all others have failed—so why not use them from the beginning?

Clearly, then, we are saying that for optimal functioning, the optimal interventions are those that support enhanced energy flows in the body and minimize interruptions of those flows. The methods outlined in Part Three are a step into the unlimited potential of Era III medicine for restoring health and well-being in all circumstances and for all conditions.

References

Achterberg, Jeanne. *Imagery in Healing*. Boston: Shambhala, 1985.

A Course in Miracles. Wisconsin Dells, WI: A Course in Miracles International, 2005.

Cousins, Norman. *Anatomy of an Illness as Perceived by the Patient*. New York: Penguin, 1981.

Dossey, Larry. *Healing Words: The Power of Prayer and the Practice of Medicine*. New York: HarperCollins, 1993.

———. *Reinventing Medicine*. New York: HarperCollins, 1999.

Gerber, Richard. *Vibrational Medicine*. Santa Fe, NM: Bear, 1988.

Jacobson, Edmund. *Progressive Relaxation*. Chicago: University of Chicago Press, 1938.

Jampolsky, Gerald. *Teach Only Love*. Hillsboro, OR: Beyond Words, 1992.

Jung, Carl G. *Memories, Dreams, Reflections: Life After Death*. New York: Random House, 1961.

Lawlis, G. Frank. *Transpersonal Medicine*. Boston: Shambhala, 1996.

Murphy, Michael. *The Future of the Body*. Los Angeles: Tarcher, 1992.

Myss, Caroline. *The Anatomy of the Spirit*. New York: Harmony Books, 1994.

Schlitz, Marilyn, et al. *Consciousness and Healing*. St. Louis, MO: Elsevier, 2005.

Sogyal Rinpoche. *The Tibetan Book of Living and Dying*. New York: HarperCollins, 1994.

Targ, Russell, and Jane Katra. *Miracles of Mind*. Novato, CA: New World Library, 1999.

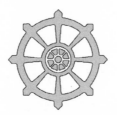

PART THREE

Healing Methods

CHAPTER 7

Cardio-Awareness
Healing Systems

WESTERN ERA I MEDICINE has operated on the assumption that the heart is an organ with a single purpose: to pump blood through the body. Recent research, however, has revealed that the heart is the primary element in a complex system of psycho-emotional and physiological interactions.

Over the past decade, research has revealed that the heart is a highly complex, self-organized information-processing center with its own functional nerve-center, or "mini-brain." The more research is completed, the more apparent it is that the heart continuously communicates with the brain and body through a variety of channels, including the nervous system, hormonal system, and many bioelectromagnetic interactions. In a single human heart cycle, blood pressure influences the brain and all the central nervous system electrically, through a baro-receptor system, converting blood pressure into neural impulses.

The rate of information change in a single heart cycle seems to be indicative of the heart's influence on the nerve cells. The messages that the heart sends to the brain not only affect physiological regulation, they influence perception, emotions, behaviors, performance, and health. In addition, the heart generates a powerful electromagnetic field that acts as a basis for all internal fields and extends out infinitely from the body.

According to the Institute of HeartMath (IHM) materials:

Research on the heart as an energetic system examines the heart's field as a carrier of emotional information and a mediator of bioelectromagnetic communication both within and outside the body. This research has shown that our heart's field changes distinctly as we experience different emotions, is registered by the brains of people around us, and also appears to be capable of affecting cells, water, and DNA studied in vitro. The implications of these findings are that people may be capable of affecting their environment in ways not previously understood, and that such "energetic" interactions may be prominently influenced by our emotions. Growing evidence also suggests that energetic interactions involving the heart may underlie intuition and important aspects of human consciousness. (Institute of HeartMath website: www.heartmath.org)

With this kind of information, we can visualize the heart as an extensive electrical interface with all mind-body systems, both internal and external.

IHM, through their Heart Research Center, has documented evidence that the heart plays an important role in the generation and perception of emotion. Based on this research, IHM has developed and tested tools and techniques to elicit what they call "physiological coherence," characterized by increased efficiency, order, and harmony in the overall functioning of the mind-body system, and associated with improved emotional stability and cognitive performance. This mode is induced through a program of self-awareness, supported by biofeedback technologies and other training modes. Techniques are applied that increase coherence in rhythmic patterns of heart rate variability, with results that include shifts in perception and the ability to reduce stress and deal more effectively with difficult situations.

These and other research results have led to the development of a new, systems-oriented model of emotion. This new model includes the heart, the brain, and the nervous and hormonal systems as components of a dynamic, interactive network from which emotional experience emerges and through which we affect all of our body and environment. Such a model suggests that a deeper experience of the heart and its rhythms can have a significant effect on the harmonious well-being of the individual.

Audio-Biofeedback

ONE OF THE MOST PROFOUND EXPERIENCES made possible by modern technology is to be immersed in one's own heart sound, to calm and heal the mind-body by relaxing into the rhythm of one's own heart. Just as the intentional shift from mind to awareness that we call meditation is calming, the intentional shift from mind to heart calms both the mind and the heart. This method uses the heart as an entrance-point into mind-body awareness and healing—hence the name, cardio-awareness healing.

The first development of a cardio-awareness healing system was the collaborative effort of the developers of harmonic compression technology from Bell Labs, a director of Columbia Records, and Robert Newman of Gain Ground during the years 1968–70. The systems were tested at Gain Ground in New York City in November 1968, and at the University of California at San Diego (UCSD) in May 1969.[17]

Since then, a whole body of research and practical tools have been developed around the heart rate as a basic rhythm, notably Sheila Ostrander and Lynn Schroeder's *Superlearning* (1994), which encourages the use of background music based on fifty to sixty

---

17. Systems development: Robert Newman, Gain Ground. Electronics: Philips Electronics Corp. Sound engineering: Norman Dolph, Columbia Records. Harmonic compression: Bell Labs, New Jersey.

beats a minute to enhance mental capacity, and the work of the Institute of HeartMath, which began with a focus on the rhythm of the heart as a foundation for all mind-body processes.

In 1995 a group of high-anxiety women were given wristwatch heart monitors so they could observe their pulse. The women were asked to observe the monitors for ten minutes a day. After twelve weeks, these women saw immediate dips in daily anxiety and also significant long-term changes in their anxiety. *Prevention* magazine called this regular observation "meditation without the meditation" (Munson 1996).

The original cardio-awareness system was developed to test the hypothesis that the mind-quieting effects of hearing one's own heart beat, amplified, may help people concentrate and maintain healing present-moment awareness better than traditional, nontechnological methods. In various meditation methods, attention is brought to the body, particularly to the breath, as a way of focusing and calming into the present moment and shifting out of ordinary reality. If focusing attention into the body was known to have such benefits, focusing on biological rhythms should have a similar mind-calming and awareness-enhancing effect, with corresponding hormonal benefits.

To experience the first cardio-awareness system, in New York and at UCSD, dozens of people at a time waited for their turn to be immersed in the sound of their own heart beat. They waited in a preparatory room listening to different recordings of the sound of the human heart in states of calm, encouraging a psychic shift to a state in which the mind was quiet and awareness was optimal. Then they were guided one by one into the round red audio chamber, the hub of the system. Once inside, they were assisted by two helpful attendants who were silent and respectful. One by one, people were seated in the "throne," a transformed dentist's chair with audio-system controls concealed behind it. They were in a relaxed posture, deep in the reclining chair. The concept behind the "throne" was that the power and majesty of each person's biological force was being respected and revealed, in an atmosphere that was calming and relaxing.

A velvet cloth was placed on the chest, and the participant's hands were folded over it. Nothing was said. Unknown to the person, under their hands and over their heart was a sensitive electronic stethoscope, connected to a high quality sound system.

The sound system was adjusted very carefully to each individual, to ensure that people were not overwhelmed by their heart sound. The sound level and clarity allowed for spontaneous immersion in that person's own coronary power. The guides receded into the background after facilitating each stage of the audio-biofeedback program.

The First Stage of Immersion: Audio-Biofeedback (via speakers in the walls of the round room)

In the first stage of cardio-entrance induced calm awareness (which is, in fact, a form of meditation), the participant is seated in the cardio-immersion throne, holding the sensitive electronic microphone in place over his or her own heart without knowing that it is concealed in the red cloth under his or her hands. The nurse attendants are now behind the chair, managing the concealed audio-controls. Soon the participant hears his or her own heart beat coming from four speakers inside the red satin walls of the chamber, hearing clearer than they have ever heard their heart. There's an immediate sense that the listener's awareness affects the heart energy, offering a coherent mind-body experience, typically calming, inducing a healthy respect for the miracle of normal function, and a sense that mind, on some level, must be everywhere in the body. This induces a healing appreciation, enhancing well-being.

The Second Stage of Immersion: Harmonic Compression Instruction to Help Hear the Sound (via mix in headphones)

Placing headphones over the ears, the attendants adjust the controls so that in one ear the participant hears audio-guidance, from a voice accelerated through harmonic compression, and in the other ear, his or her own live heart sound. The accelerated hearing lets the participant hear the instructions for cardio-immersion, and know them, twice as fast. The mix of the two provides a simultaneous entry into the biological richness of the heart sound with the accelerated voice, encouraging a deeper hearing and increasing the healing potential.

> The fundamental pulsations of the body are particularly fruitful to focus on during meditation because they are so intimately connected with the experience of being alive. (Kabat-Zinn 1990, 48)

The Third Stage of Immersion: Audio-Biofeedback (via speakers in the walls of the round room)

After the first calming immersion in the participant's heart beat, and after the instructions have been heard in harmonic compression, the third phase of hearing the energy of one's own heart builds on the calming of the first two phases, enhancing both heart and immune function through simply listening to the sound of one's own heart in the headphones. Self-calming meditation reduces blood pressure, slows heart rate, balances heart arrhythmia, and lowers cortisol levels that restrict immune function.

Audio-Visual Transform

THE EFFECTIVENESS of the audio-biofeedback system just described led to the development of a new cardio-therapy and diagnostic system in 1970.[18] This second system transformed heart sound into dynamic images of the heart beat, via oscilloscope technology, which could be used diagnostically and therapeutically at once. The use of an electronic stethoscope with sophisticated oscilloscope capability produces heart activity information for diagnosis and research.

The images presented here are recordings of one human heart cycle. As experienced in live biofeedback, each image contains the subject's awareness in a healing immersion. The sound and imagery of the fourfold spiral contraction are shown in live spiral lines of sound. The image is unique and unrepeatable yet has definite diagnostic value. It's conducive to the experience of the preciousness of every moment of life, which is healing in the same way that meditation is, bringing us back from the obstructions caused by normal mind activity.

Heart activity can be readily made visible by current technology. The images here are images from an oscilloscope. When cardio images are projected on a screen by laser

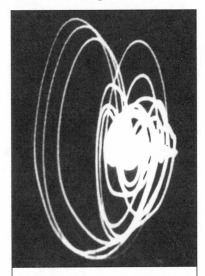

Figure 3. Cardio-awareness: one unrepeatable heart cycle. Oscilloscope image: innermost loops are low frequency.

18. System development: Robert Newman, Gain Ground. System design and realization: Ted Wolff, NYU Medical Center Research.

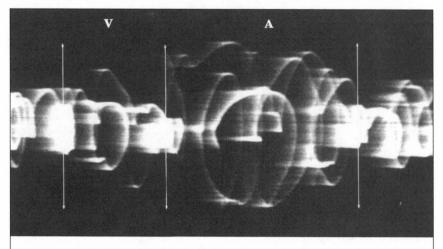

Figure 4. Vital charge of information. In this live oscilloscope image of one complete heart cycle, the V indicates contractions in the ventricles and the A indicates contractions in the auricles.

technology in live biofeedback, the system offers a dynamic potential for health enhancement and diagnosis through bio-immersion.

References

Kabat-Zinn, Jon. *Full Catastrophe Living*. New York: Bantam-Doubleday Dell, 1990.

Munson, Marty. "The Easy Road: Monitoring Pulse Rate May Bring About Reduction in Stress." *Prevention* (March 1996): 25–26.

Ostrander, Sheila, and Lynn Schroeder. *Superlearning*. New York: Bantam-Doubleday Dell, 1994.

CHAPTER 8

Progressive
Neuromuscular Release

THERE ARE MANY RELAXATION THERAPIES in the field of mind-body medicine (MBM). Furthermore, relaxation is often an element of other MBM techniques such as meditation, hypnosis, yoga, and so forth. Nonetheless, there is one relaxation technique that stands out and has been extensively studied: progressive muscle relaxation. Originally developed by Edmund Jacobson (1938), it was in its original form a technique requiring dozens of sessions wherein the subject was taught to relax approximately thirty different muscle groups (Barrows and Jacobs 2001).

Throughout a distinguished clinical and research career at the Harvard Medical School and then at the University of Chicago Medical School, from the 1930s through the 1940s, Dr. Jacobson developed many Progressive Relaxation (PR) techniques, from isometric exercises for specific muscle groups, to total system methods. The object of all the methods was to release neuromuscular stresses on the nervous system in order to treat nervous system conditions corresponding to various disease conditions. "Because of reflex connections, the nervous system cannot be quieted except in conjunction with the muscular system" (Jacobson 1938, xii). "The neuromuscular factor as a cause and element of the symptomatology of various disease processes has seemed evident" (ibid., 430).

Through releasing specific muscular system stresses on the nervous system he was able to treat the nervous system correspondences to many disease conditions and reverse the basis of those conditions. "Relaxation evidently applies to a larger field of disorders, since various conditions in internal medicine which are not psychogenic come within its scope" (ibid., 429).

Nervous hypertension with fatigability ("neurasthenia") is a widespread condition, characterized by nervous tension and various associated disorders, often with the inability to sit still. Jacobson's isometric and whole-body relaxation procedures helped the mind-body calm down therapeutically. Some of his methods were sitting practices, and many were reclining, but they all made people stop and alter their function by themselves.

> In the treatment of nervous states, ... there is increasing evidence that the subsidence of symptoms becomes most marked upon the disappearance of residual tensions. (ibid., 15)

Integral to Jacobson's work was Sir William Osler's knowledge of the use of rest in medicine (Osler 1932). Rest and self-care, shifting responsibility to the patient, were the basis of a breakthrough in therapeutic direction. The emphasis in treatment programs shifted from care in the medical office to home care. "The aim of nervous system treatment will be to point out to the patient the voluntary element in these symptoms and to guide him to rid himself of them" (Jacobson 1938, 406).

When Jacobson imparted his methods to his patients, he made it clear that it was essential that the patients apply the methods regularly at home as self-care. In fact, Jacobson was the first published medical practitioner developing methods in which self-care would be emphasized. He anticipated the potential for self-care in a new era of medicine, and so he initiated the new paradigm and gave it effective mind-body methods.

Jacobson's system was simplified by Douglas Bernstein and Thomas Borovec (1973), and since then, other professionals have modified his methods even further. In 1979 Jon Kabat-Zinn introduced Jacobson's full-body PR in a forty-five-minute "body scan" integral to the groundbreaking program at UMMC, and, through the UMMC program, added a new dimension to Jacobson's method, making it more efficient and even more effective: mindfulness meditation.

The time-honored method of mindfulness meditation, a method by which people are able to control attention and maintain focus in spite of the disturbances of the mind, made PR more effective than ever. Patients and doctors have identified the following benefits of mindfulness meditation with PR, among others:

- relaxation of the conceptual, logical mind

- self-regulated attention (focus)

- self-induced state (self-care)

- muscle relaxation

With the addition of mindfulness, PR becomes more complete. Instead of being limited by disturbances of the mind, the practice becomes awareness-enhanced.

In 1997 MediGrace, a nonprofit corporation established to expand the use of meditation in medicine,[19] further developed mindfulness-based PR to give it even greater potential in both preventing and reversing disease conditions. The essential feature added by MediGrace is specific direction to engage life force on a cellular level. Since 1997 MediGrace has used its modification of mindfulness-based PR in more than eighty hospital trainings, with the support of the California Board of Registered Nursing. More than a thousand patients have used the method in their self-care programs. The practice that follows is a version of the script offered in the MediGrace audio-guide.

---

19. MediGrace was originally founded by Robert Newman as the World Health Foundation in New York and is now located in Southern Oregon. More information can be found by searching the website: www.medigrace.org.

Advanced Progressive Relaxation:
Practice of Deep Release

L IKE MEDITATION, PR IS DEPENDENT upon regular and sincere daily practice. If that is done, then many adverse conditions are treatable by PR. It treats the whole health condition, through the nerves and the mind. For an age of nervous system challenges, PR is a needed mind-body medicine.

Advanced PR uses the body scan procedure, accelerating healing in several ways:

- People see that with the method they can make shifts into better function through self-care.

- People are brought by this self-care procedure to a new state of consciousness, free of conditions.

- People are guided to engage life force on the cellular level.

- People experience inner light, which experience has been shown to enhance inner harmony and well-being.

These factors work together in the procedure of *Practice of Deep Release*, a forty-five-minute reclining PR meditation indicated for most disorders and adverse conditions.

The following three methods—*Practice of Deep Release, Breathing Healing Energy,* and *Reversal of Suffering*—are presented here in versions of the methods available in audio-guide transmission on the Calm Healing CD (MG3). With this CD, you can experience the methods in privacy, with concentration, for the full benefits.

THE METHOD

❧

Practice of Deep Release

Introduction

This practice is for anyone who needs energy and healing.
It's done lying down.
It's really good for nervousness and stress.
You get pain management and optimal function.
You get a new sense of body and vitality.
In this practice you slowly go through your whole body and
   relax it, patiently.
You save energy and you gain new energy as you enter new
   resources.
The energy increase is essential for healing and it brings calm.
It will take about forty-five minutes to go through the process.

Find yourself a comfortable place to lie down.
If you're bedridden, lie flat on your back and straighten your
   body if you can.
If you're able to lie down on the floor, a mat or blankets or a rug
   is ideal for doing this practice.
The effects of this practice are immediate and they also build up
   over time.
The most benefits come from doing it every day.
It's a direct way of relaxing into energy and healing.
Make sure that you're going to be warm enough, and lie down
   mindfully.
Be aware that you're not lying down to take a nap and avoid
   falling asleep.
Keep your eyes open and softly focused.
You may close your eyes briefly from time to time to rest them
   and to see into life inside, but keep your eyes open as much as
   possible.

As much as you do the deep release practice
you come into your potential more and more.
Be patient with this practice.
Be patient with yourself.
Especially if you're suffering a chronic condition with physical or
    mental pain,
do this practice again and again, to relax the tensions caused by
    the pain,
to come fresh into the next moment of life.
Stay in your living presence.
This practice is designed to make you confident, energized, and
    calm.
The energy you will feel works directly to make you well.

The Practice ·

When you're ready, take a deep breath and then exhale easily.
Begin feeling the sensation of life energy working in all your
    body at once.
Take another deep breath,
deep into life,
and breathe out the release your systems need for optimal
    function.

As if you're doing it for the first time, come into your whole body
    at once.
Feel the trillions of cells and energy flows.
Let yourself feel all the sensations of having a live human body.
There's so much life in it, it's inconceivable—
ten trillion living cells,
all working together to create a force of life in you.
When you feel your whole body directly,
it feels like unlimited life.
Keep feeling the sensation of all the life currents,
the many electric body processes.

Feel all the life going on in you at once.
Feel the cohesion into flesh.

As you become aware of life itself in you, just relax into that.
Let go of pain,
again and again and again.
Let go of suffering again and again.
Let go of any tensions or constrictions.
You're going to take this time to relax yourself all the way
    through,
slowly but surely.

Soon you will focus part by part through your body,
feeling all the life in it at once.
You go through your body,
from your feet to your head,
to take muscle pressure off your nerves.
For the sake of your nerves
you need to release unconscious tension in all muscle systems.

Stay in touch with the sensation of life in your whole body,
from the crown down.
Starting with the toes of your left foot,
feel all the life in your toes.
Feel the functions of the bones—
all that they always do that you don't notice.
Feel the channels of energy that run through your feet.
Feel how it all works together.
Feel your toes and all of your foot vibrating together.
Feel how much life there is in it.
If there is any tension or pain,
locate exactly where,
and relax the muscles and tendons there.
Let them open into the total current.

Feel in your foot all the work it has been doing for your body all
    these years.
Relax any clenched muscles or tension in your tendons.
Open whatever needs to be opened.
Relax it into its open-and-ready state.
There may be muscles and tendons that haven't relaxed for years.
You are there inside them, so just let them open.
Feel how this benefits your arteries and your nerves.

Bring your attention from your left foot into your left ankle.
Feel all the energy flows going through it, to and from all parts of
    your body.
Find and open any tight muscle or tendon.
Let your ankle relax into its softness, pliant and able.
Feel the goodness of the electrical flow,
the goodness of the blood flow,
and the connection with all the life flows in your body.
Know them now.

Let your awareness move up into the calf of your left leg.
Feel all the muscles in your calf.
Be aware of all the work these muscles do in helping you
    maintain your life.
Appreciate that.
Have a good feeling for what is there, and then relax it.
Let it open.
Let your flesh and bone optimize its aliveness.
All throughout your foot and lower leg,
feel, relax, and open all the muscles you can find.
Find them all.
Relax them all.
Relax anything that feels like tension in the nerves of your lower
    leg.
Feel healed and whole throughout your lower leg and foot.

Now go up through your left knee.
Feel all the sensation in your knee.
This is such a simple way to meditate, going through your body,
knowing your body as if for the first time.
Let your body save energy and heal by opening and coming
    alive.

Come up into your left thigh.
Feel how your thigh supports your body in life.
Feel its energy
and release any tension that's there.
Effortlessly, relax all you can throughout your entire left leg.
There may be tensions there that haven't been relaxed for years.
Just find them.
You're there inside them.
All throughout your leg and foot feel the big muscles and the
    small ones.
Feel it all together.
And relax it all together.
Feel a relaxing and healing in your nerves.
Feel your blood flow with all the wonderful work it does.
Feel all the life flow sensation.
Open into it all.
Rest into it all.

Now begin to notice your right foot.
Feel the toes of your right foot.
Feel all the life in each toe.
Continue to feel your whole left leg.
The life current of that is with you as you go through your right
    leg.
Everything you've brought your attention to is still in your
    awareness

as you go through more and more of your body,
releasing tensions and shifting function.
You unlock and unblock,
taking care of your own needs,
taking out the basis of any harmful condition,
coming to the basis of new life.

In your right foot, contact all the bones and the life-fields.
Through the ball of your foot and the arch,
feel all the work your foot does for you.
Feel all the life service in your foot.
On its sensitive sole,
feel the endpoints of energy channels of your body—
the points recognized by various medical traditions.
Now feel the importance of those energy points on the bottoms
    of both your feet, connected to all the functions of your body.
Feeling the energy of these endpoints helps you start to clear any
    harmful conditions.
You can let go of old patterns affecting the nervous system,
releasing the nerves for new function.

Come up through your right ankle,
relaxing it,
come up into the calf of your right leg,
feeling all of its flesh and bone.
Find and open all the muscles in your calf,
releasing any constricted flows.
Heal into fresh life energy.
Open more of anything needing to be opened in your legs.
Release more and more of any tensions blocking the full flow of
    life
in the flesh and in the bone.
Feel the life sensations all at once.
You are it all.

You can feel it all.
Know it all.
Relax whatever may be habitually tense.
Feel the energy gain in relaxing.

Come up from your right calf through all the sensation in your
    knee,
into your thigh.
In an enlivening way you're coming through more and more of
    your body.
You have an unused resource to heal into.
You have to let go to heal into it.
The sensation of all the life in us at once is available all the time,
but unless you give it attention you live without its benefits.

The most benefits come from practicing every day.
Becoming still and letting go of movement,
we heal into the total sensation of deep body.
It's the body of life free of all conditioning,
the basis of wholeness and healing.

Throughout the duration of this meditation practice,
build your strength of connection with fresh body.
Now, in your right thigh,
throughout all its muscles and tendons,
blood vessels and nerves,
there's a growing sense of ease.
If any pain or tension persists,
breathe into and out of the pain and tension.
Feel how muscles tighten all around pain in resistance,
trying to block it out.
Relax the muscle resistance
and accommodate the pain or tension.
Breathe it in and give it space.

The key is not to identify with the pain.
Breathe into and out of that area if you need to at any time,
but keep with the direction of this practice,
continuing to enter unused life.

Relax more and more,
in greater awareness,
with your nerves working in a more healed way.
Come from your thighs up through your loins into your belly:
your navel and solar plexus power centers.
Feel the whole lower half of your body,
from your abdomen down.
Feel all the life and life support in it.

Now once again, feel your whole body,
deeper and more completely than ever.
Feel all the dynamics of your central nervous system,
taking care of billions of functions at once.
Feel the energy of all your higher systems,
silently performing countless activities,
ingeniously working,
ceaselessly working for greater life.
Feel that you embody the realization of life.
You were born to have and experience this all.
It's time to be what you really are:
a body inconceivably alive.

Breathe into any areas of pain or tension.
Welcome the sensations of your body's tension and pain,
to come into the greater life you have.
Staying relaxed in your abdomen and breathing there,
see wonderful living systems in yourself.
Since they are yours,
you can know them,

and enter the bliss of all the life at work in you,
life flowing in all the channels of your potential.
See the light of all the electrical flows.
See the bodies of light in your cells.
Heal your pains into the unity of that light.

Now in your abdomen and your solar plexus
feel any tensions collected there over the years.
Stay in your navel, breathing easily and deeply.
You are there, inside,
and now your attention is in there too.
You know your own gut area.
Open more and more of all the holding,
all the resisting.
Let go more and more of the results of your habitual actions and
    your impending actions.
Relax it all.
Free yourself completely from actions.
Free yourself from the stress and activity of life.
Free yourself from the built-up tensions of your lifetimes.
Free yourself to relax into your being, your unconditioned life.
In stillness, and in peace, heal into it.

Relax every small and large muscle in your belly and solar plexus.
Feel how that enhances the relaxing of your nerves for greater
    function.
Come up into your upper body.
Relax all the musculature throughout your chest.
Find any muscles contracted or partly contracted throughout
    your rib cage,
and around your ribs.
Feel any collected tension in your chest.
Release all tension from within.
You can do it.

Spontaneously relax it all from within.
Open your chest and shoulders,
breathing in deeply,
and relaxing as you exhale and release.
Come into your heart area.
Enter the dynamic majesty of your heartwork.
Be thankful that it runs itself so well.
Appreciate its power,
and how every cell in your body helps it beat.
Be all the light of the electricity in its beats.
Feel the gift of miracles within miracles making all this life flow.
See that the powerful blood-beat is full of your light.
See your body-light in all your systems.
Feel with the full force of your embodiment that you are healing
    in all this life.
The very presence of all this life in you is your healing.

Now feel your whole back.
Feel whatever tensions there may be in the spine.
Where gravity and personal tensions have been compressing or
    fusing vertebrae,
let that stop.
Let the bone spontaneously unlock.
Let your whole spine open.
Feel its bones and nerves adjust, ready to come to life.

Come up your spine, through your shoulders,
and into your neck.
Open, and let sensation flow.
The tension of daily living can lock the head and spine.
Spontaneously unlock it from within.
It could seem difficult,
but simply unlock the built-up tensions of your upper body and
    neck.

Feel the natural ease of releasing any excessive contractions
throughout your back and neck and head.
Open the muscles.
Feel the energy gain.
Let it flow, enlivening you with new functions.
Relax all the muscles around your head,
muscles connecting your head to your neck and shoulders.
Relax in the awareness that comes alive when important life
    energy is gained.
From head to toe,
feel the cohesion of coming together
in total flow of life sensation.

If you want to flow instead of wasting energy in unconscious
    tensions,
feel how natural it is to be at ease in deep release.
Check your head and neck for any remaining tension.
Save energy,
letting any holding unfold.
Let it all melt down.
Time to let it be naturally open.
Feel the total field of the muscular complexity of your body.
Feel how good it would be to completely open it.
You can do that.
Come into your face now, starting with your jaw.
Breathe into it and let your jaw loosen,
now completely letting go of the need to speak.
All throughout your lower face,
feel any muscular tension,
and relax it.
Give your jaw a chance to really rest,
to save your energy,
and your teeth.
Start reversing any tension in your mouth.

Let it be in its natural ease.
Feel all the different sets of muscles in your mouth,
forming your expressions,
conscious and unconscious.
Find all those muscles,
and relax them.
Release all the residual expression
and the tendency to expression.
Let yourself be free of that now.
Relax into a state where you are free of active tendencies,
free in your unconditioned body,
free in your unconditioned life.
Relax your jaw,
your mouth,
and your cheeks.
Relax your entire lower face
into the total sensation of life energy.
Feel all habitual patterns dissolving in greater awareness.

Now feel all the muscles connected to your eyes,
forming the expression in and around them,
habitual and spontaneous expression,
all that you know as yourself.
Move carefully through all your eye muscles,
relaxing that musculature more and more.
Move carefully through the muscles around your right eye.
Relax any tension you find.
Now go through all the muscles around your left eye.
Relax them.
Release all the potential of expression around both your eyes.
Let your eyes rest in themselves.

Feeling yourself becoming free,
relax into the free body of life that you are.

Rest free of all external activity now,
and free of conscious and unconscious mind.
Rest free of any harmful conditioning in your body channels and
   pathways.
Feel like you're coming alive for the first time.
Rest in freedom from life and death.
From your eyes come up into your brows and forehead.
Feel your forehead muscles latent with expressions.
Now, consciously,
throughout your forehead,
relax any overt or subtle expression.
Relax into your inherent open awareness,
free of life and death.

Now feel both your arms at once,
flowing with life.
Feel all the life expression in your arms and hands.
Feel the life energies in the fingers of both hands.
Feel life force throughout your fingers and hands.
Feel the inherent healing capability in your hands.
Feel all the vital channels in your wrists.
Relax any subtle tensions in your hands and wrists.
More and more,
feel the bliss of normal function in your body,
as if coming into it with awareness for the first time.

Feel your forearms
and come up through your elbows
into your upper arms.
Feel the activity potential of your arms and hands.
Feel the blessing and goodness of that.
Feel all of both arms at once,
relaxing all the tendencies into the activities of life
to come to it all afresh.

Relax in inaction.
Free yourself from the actions of body,
speech,
and mind.
Enter the deathless energy of greater awareness.

And now again,
know your multidimensional body of life all at once,
more in contact than you've ever been with your greater life.
Heal into that greater life.
Come to it more and more.
See that it is unlimited.
It is your unlimited potential.
Use this practice to come to life, again and again.
Feel how natural it is to feel well.
Open your body—
nerve and muscle—
every day.
Let yourself feel the healing
and the life energy gain.

The more you give to the practice,
the more you heal.
Feeling more and more at ease in deep release,
feel all your systems flowing with life.
Resting in inaction,
you come in a fresh way to your potential.

Do this practice to calm your mind, which causes so much tension.
If you're patient and persevering, you'll see that mind can be
calmed. Follow this procedure. Again and again come through your
whole body, resting free of the basis of any harmful conditions.

In ending this practice, break stillness with awareness. See how
much you can be aware of timelessness as you move.

References

Barrows, Kevin A., and Bradly P. Jacobs. "Mind-Body Medicine: An Introduction and Review of the Literature," draft, September 2001.

Bernstein, Douglas, and Thomas Borovec. *Progressive Relaxation Training: A Manual for the Helping Professions.* Champaign, IL: Research Press, 1973.

Jacobson, Edmund. *Progressive Relaxation.* Chicago: University of Chicago Press, 1938.

Kabat-Zinn, Jon. *Full-Catastrophe Living.* New York: Bantam-Doubleday, 1990.

Osler, Sir William. *Aequanimitas,* 2nd ed. New York: McGraw-Hill, 1932.

CHAPTER 9

Awareness-Based
Energy Breathing

IN MANY OF THE GREAT MASTER PATHS developed over human history, breathing energy into the navel center is the heart of the practice. In *Tai Chi*, one is directed to "sink the *chi* into the *Tan Tien*," the *Tan Tien* being near the center of the navel. In *Zen* meditation, one breathes into the *Hara*, the vital center just below the center of the navel. In *Vajrayana* meditation, one breathes into the Life Vase, *Tse Bum* (Tibetan), the Vase of Immortality, centered between four finger widths above the naval and four finger widths below the navel. In all traditions the benefits have been cited as increased vitality and longevity. With respect to health care today, the benefits are multidimensional.

Vase-Breathing Meditation

AWARENESS-BASED ENERGY BREATHING is called, in Tibetan, *Bum Chung* or Vase Breathing. In this form of meditation, breathwork is transformative. The focus of the practice is on the natural, uncontrived movement of breathing through which energy flows into the energy body. In general, awareness of and identification with breathing is the calming basis of the return to the fundamental awareness, the basis of the shift out of the disorder of the mind.

Staying with the breath, no matter how the mind tries to seduce your attention, is transformative in itself. In the Vase Breathing practice, awareness becomes energy breathing, and in sustained conscious energy breathing is the power to transform, to heal and evolve. In mindfulness meditation, body is ordinary and breathing is ordinary—profound but ordinary. In Vase Breathing, body is extraordinary and breathing is extraordinary. In many therapeutic methods, breathing in the belly and centering awareness there are important as a practical discipline. With Vase Breathing, there is a radically different sense of the body and its breathing capability, plus a radically different sense of air and the field of life. In mindfulness meditation, the belly is the center of gravity of the body, and belly breathing lowers one's center of cognitive function. In Vase Breathing, we learn that there is an important breathing feature in our energy body, the Life Vase in our navel center, and that in the air we breathe is a breathable energy that sustains life, called *prana* or *chi*. In ordinary deep breathing, which is certainly healthy, air is understood to be the source of oxygen vital to life. In Vase Breathing one breathes oxygen and energy into a body of subtle energy systems, each with its own energetic features.

As a result, Vase Breathing becomes a dual means of healing. The more one shifts from mind into awareness, the more one realizes the radiant nature of the *rigpa,* awareness itself, the inner luminosity, free of obstruction; the more one experiences the nature of awareness, the more one is able to release any mind-body disorders. With Vase Breathing we simultaneously breathe energy into the energy body for greater function while resting in the inner light of *rigpa.*

What is the Vase? The Tibetan word *bum,* vase, is a central element of energy body anatomy. As we explored earlier, the inner or energy body component of human embodiment is characterized by numerous energy channels and systems, around a central energy channel (CEC). The CEC has a vertical series of power centers or *chakras* (wheels), rising to the crown *chakra*. In the Tibetan tradition of *Bum Chung,* the vertical series of *chakras* aligned in the CEC arise from the bottom of an energy form called the Vase of Immortality, the base of the CEC, in the navel center.

The perennial wisdom is that we are born with a capacity to breathe energies vital to our realization of life and greater health. In the UMMC program, people are directed to "breathe into" interior areas of their body. Breath is not spoken of as energy, but it is assumed that we can energetically intend or direct "breath" into internal areas of the body. In Vase Breathing, we use imagery to move energy from the air down into the Vase, from which it moves up into the CEC, to harmonize or "balance" the operation of the subtle energy power centers, bringing higher systems to life.

So how exactly do we breathe and utilize the energy around us?

Vase Breathing is visualization-enhanced breathing. In Vase Breathing it is important to consciously sense the vital energy in the air and to know that we are born to breathe that energy into an energy body feature in the navel center. We intend and send that energy into a receptive soft energetic Vase in the energy body, to come into higher orders of function.

Recognizing that we have been breathing subtle energy in and out since birth without using that energy, we begin to sense and intentionally absorb it. By intending the universal energy into the navel breathing facility, our intention directs the energy into the Vase. By cultivating our inherent ability to sense and absorb the subtle energy in the air, we learn to strengthen the life force behind the immune system. The energy is absorbed into the Vase directly from the air in the lungs. It doesn't need to go into and through the blood to enter the body's systems. It is absorbed directly into the legendary Vase in the navel center, from which it moves through the central energy channel to enter and enrich every aspect of the mind-body system. And because Vase Breathing is a practice of optimizing the functions of the radiant energy body, it is a perfect practice to realize the healing luminous nature of awareness.

The profound psychological shift from mind to awareness is

identical in both mindfulness meditation and in Vase Breathing, so that both practices can be called *Vipashyana* (Insight) meditation, but Vase Breathing can also work on unconscious levels, similar to the experience called "lucid dreaming," bringing the mind-body to higher and higher levels of function. And Vase Breathing offers the experience of body and awareness as light.

Such deep, Vase Breathing sitting meditation supports a five-fold energy gain.

1. By sitting and calming down, people save energy that would have been lost in general activity. People relax.

2. Meditation is better than sleep for restoring energy reserves; the calm state is less disturbing than the dream state.

3. People save energy that would have been lost in the ceaseless activity of the mind. By shifting from mind to awareness, people drop mind and save important mind-body energy.

4. People generally breathe with inefficient, high chest, or inter-costal respiration, which burns up as much as seven times more energy than deep breathing. Vase Breathing saves people from wasting energy in the wrong breathing.

5. People who breathe energy into their energy bodies experience greater vitality and well-being.

These benefits make it clear that a meditation method using this inherent optimal breathing facility can be a significant medical method.

This method offers people maximum oxygenation plus vital energies, and experience of inner light, as a means for transforming the mind-body.

THE METHOD

Breathing Healing Energy

Introduction

There are two elements: what breathes and what is breathed.
You see that you have an important breathing Vase in your navel
    center,
a Vase made to breathe energies of the universal field.
You sense that you were born to breathe vital energy.
You visualize the radiant energetic activity of your body
with your brilliant *chakra* power centers and other energy body
    features.
So what is breathed is energy medicine in the air,
and what breathes is a deep-breathing body of light.

In the beginning, do this sitting practice for fifteen or twenty
    minutes each time.
And do the practice at least once a day.
If possible use cushions and sit on the floor.
If you have pain or discomfort, sit in a chair with your spine
    balanced upright.
If you're bedridden, cushions or pillows can help you raise your
    back as upright as possible.
It's not the spine so much as the central psychic channel that's
    being held upright
to help you to greater awareness and greater function.

The Practice

Sit down into your whole body,
or sit up into your whole body,
and get the sensation of all the life in you at once.
Feel it.
Feel the aliveness in the stillness.
Adjust your body a little if you need to.

You should be relaxed and alert,
feeling stable and balanced.

See how that helps you feel well.
Keep coming back to the sensation
of all the energy currents moving in your body at once.
See how that feels like a direct experience of healing.

By being quiet and still,
you come into that.
It's always there.
Every moment you come back to it
it's like a moment of instant healing.

You are going to breathe in a new way.
Both the way you breathe and what you breathe will be
    extraordinary,
but completely natural,
not forcing your breathing at all.

Breathe with your belly.
Practice natural abdominal breathing, easy and deep.
Imagine that your whole body of nervous and psychic pathways
    is full of light.
And inside your navel area
there is a luminous Vase you breathe into.

In Chinese meditation this is called the *Tan Tien*.
In *Vajrayana* meditation it's called the Vase of Life.
The practice of breathing vital essence into the Vase
increases life span and vitality.
So we sit and keep the vision of our body being full of light
and having a special breathing purpose.
Maybe for the first time in our lives

we breathe the precious energies in the air
that have always been there.
We've just never related to them.

Now we see that by relating to those vital energies in the air,
by breathing them in intentionally,
they absorb into the Vase and into the central psychic channel.

Now we see that not only do we have a special breathing Vase
    for healing the life force,
but also the medicine energies we need for healing
are in the air we've been breathing.
We've always breathed them in and out without absorbing them.
Now we're going to feed on those energies
as if they've been given to us as the perfect medicine we need
to heal into greater health and wisdom.

Get the feeling that the vital essence you need is in the air,
and you're born to breathe it,
to live on that essence.
Do it.
See that there's fine food matter in the air
and you were born to feed on it.
Breathe energy from the air into your Vase.
Please do it now.

So we're just going to sit,
as upright as possible,
comfortable and at ease,
and practice breathing vital energies
with the Vase in our bellies.
And as we do it,
without knowing what happens,
our mind may take us out of awareness.

Awareness-Based Energy Breathing

In an instant we're lost in thought.
We're no longer breathing medicine energies,
we're thinking.
We're thinking about something,
something that happened
or something that's going to happen.
You're possibly anxious about something behind the thought.
You're not present.
You're thinking and not aware of your presence.

Then something in you that wants to live wakes up.
Awareness in you that wants to be present,
an awareness that wants to be breathing vital energies,
snaps you out of the trance of thinking and wakes you up.
You come back to presence.
Keep breathing vital energy with the Vase in your belly.
See how your mind takes you away from that,
then see how you wake up,
come to,
come back to the Vase Breathing.
Please do it.

Be patient.
Be persevering to breathe in this deeper way,
this healthier way.
It helps calm you down.
It helps quiet your nerves.
You don't waste precious energy on your thinking mind.

Don't identify with your thinking mind at all
as it tries to take you out.
Stay with your Vase Breathing in open awareness.
You save the energy you'd be losing in your mind
and you take in new energies from the air you breathe.

You breathe essential energy down into the Vase,
naturally and easily,
with your abdominal muscles relaxed.
The finer matter in the air absorbs into your higher systems.
See how you save vital energy and take in vital energy by staying
    out of mind
and calming down into your body.
Please do it.

Fears may arise,
in different ways,
causing anxious thoughts.
It is very important to recognize those thoughts,
those fears.
They tend to be particularly strong in distracting you from being
    present.
It's important to recognize anxiety.
Let it be.
Let go of it,
and return to the deep breathing.
You'll see that you can do that.
If you recognize what happens in your mind and don't identify
    with it,
if you see it and free it,
you'll feel freer,
healthier,
better.
Please do it.
Breathe energy from the air into the Vase.

If you catch yourself being conscious of looking at something,
or hearing something,
just recognize that you were getting lost in that.

Expand your awareness.
Sense the light of your awareness.
Return to *deep* breathing.
Whatever comes up—
thought,
perception,
emotion—
let it arise.
See it and free it.
Calm down into your awareness.
More and more,
understand your natural ability to be free of your mind,
to be in your body in a more healed way.

Breathe free.
Feel that the energy you absorb in the Vase
may be all you need to heal with.
If you breathe this way and don't identify with what comes up in
     your mind,
you'll come into new function,
greater function.
Please do it.

Catch the thought as it comes up
and let it be free.
Don't attach to it.
Don't fix on it.
Stay in your open awareness free of your mind.
Stay with the Vase Breathing.
Do it day and night.
Do it to heal in your sleep.
Calm down to where you are present as thought happens, as it
     comes up.
Leave it alone.

It changes.
It doesn't matter what the thinking is,
let it change,
and dissolve.

Stay calm.
Don't be disturbed by or taken out by your thought.
Don't be disturbed by emotions that come up.
Stay with Vase Breathing and open awareness,
and you can be undisturbable when your fears come up.
You can be undisturbable even when death comes.

Stay with the total sensation of your body.
Feel your awareness become more alive.
Sit into life beyond life and death.
Please do it.

So train yourself in this way.
Train to use the ability you have
to stay out of the trances of your mind.
Stay in the live presence of your open awareness.

Sense all of the universe,
all of life,
present here and now.
Sense how you can come directly to life.

Just keep to the Vase Breathing and open awareness.
Stay free of mind.
Come into presence more and more.
Breathe into presence more and more.
If you have persistent pain,
breathe into and out of the pain sensations.
Relax the region of the pain more and more.

Don't let your mind make a big deal about the pain.
Breathe into it and breathe it out more and more.
See how much energy you save by coming to the pain and
    staying with it.
You prevent your own suffering.

Feel it out.
Feel the constrictions,
the resistance in the muscles around the pain.
Relax it intentionally more and more.
Breathe it in and out,
until the pain eases,
as its sensations change
and you can return to the Vase belly breathing again.

See how you save energy by working on pain directly.
When you sit into energy body,
pain sensations will change.
They may quiet down or go away.
Keep coming back to the Vase Breathing,
all the time.
Please do it.

Keep shifting into open awareness.
See the light of awareness.
This is mind-body medicine
and it's effective because you find it in yourself,
in the air so vital to your life.

It's a double medicine.
Your awareness becomes medicine
when you do such practices to improve your life quality,
and the vital energy you breathe
is great medicine.

Breathe it well.

When you come to the end of this session,
as you break stillness, do it with awareness.
You're more alive.
You've done something for your health and your life.
Let yourself do it more.

References

Chang, G. C. C. *The Six Yogas of Naropa*. Ithaca, NY: Snow Lion, 1963.

CHAPTER 10

Transformative
Compassionate Breathing

THE VARIOUS BUDDHIST TRADITIONS have given mind-body medicine some of its most useful methods, including powerful
transpersonal methods. To the thousands of Americans studying
meditation with Buddhist teachers, the practice of *Tong Len*, or
Compassionate Breathing, was an essential practice by the time
Sogyal Rinpoche published his important book, *The Tibetan Book
of Living and Dying* (1994). In the chapter called "Compassion: The
Wish-Fulfilling Jewel," the method of *Tong Len* is published with full
disclosure (Sogyal, 187ff.). In Tibetan, *Tong Len* means "Giving and
Receiving" or "Exchanging Oneself for Another." The practice has
various applications as a transpersonal healing method.

The practice of Compassionate Breathing was called the Holy
Secret. The secret is exchanging oneself for another.

Larry Dossey has documented the numerous scientific studies of
the effect of long-distance healing on others, whether or not they
know that they are being "prayed for," or that healing energy is
being intended to them (1993, 1999). Yet beyond numerous anecdotal stories, we are not aware of any clinical trials focused on the
dual healing benefits of *Tong Len*, Compassionate Breathing—studies that quantify the doubly healing benefits of the practice.

Still, Compassionate Breathing has been used in cancer care
increasingly in the past twenty years because of its effectiveness.

People can do the practice to abate their suffering and the suffering of others. A powerful use is when someone who has been lost in their suffering, say someone with AIDS or cancer, does this practice to give healing energy to another person with a similar condition. When this method is given to cancer patients or AIDS patients, enabling them to practice the healing of another patient, it's wonderful to see someone who had been dwelling in suffering shift their attention and function to practicing the healing of others.

This is what typically can happen (the following is a true story):

You are going to visit a woman dying of cancer in an oncology center. She is the mother of a friend of yours. You haven't met the woman. She knows that you're coming to visit her. She's alone in her room. She's glad that you've come. You ask her if she'd like a little massage on her neck and shoulders. She says she'd love that. She loves being caringly touched. You ask her how she is. She starts to describe her suffering. You breathe with her, in increasing communion. Then you ask her if she'd like to do some meditation. She says, yes. She's never done that but she'd like to. You say that we're going to meditate with the breath. You ask her if she knows someone suffering from cancer as badly as she is. She pauses for a moment and then says, yes, she does know someone. You ask her to say that person's name aloud. She does. You repeat the name. You say here's what we're going to do. Just forget your sickness. Part of you has always been well, has always been free. Right now, forget about being sick; just think about the person you've just mentioned. It doesn't matter how far away she is. You're going to reach that person instantly in your heart. This is more real and practical than probably anything you can imagine. You can practice the healing of that person with your breath. Just breathe naturally, focusing into the sickness and suffering of that person. On your in-breath effortlessly breathe in all you can of that person's sickness and suffering. Let it energetically come into your heart. That person's energy simply dissolves into light in your body. And effortlessly breathe out into that person all the energy they need to heal. You repeat the instruction once. You ask if she understands. She says yes. Then you do the practice together. You feel the presence of the other woman. You and your friend's mother silently practice healing that woman. After a few minutes you realize that you're in the presence of something marvelous. The dying woman you're visiting has changed. She's become the practice of healing. You continue the practice for about five minutes. It feels very powerful. You know that it's a remarkable event. The experience of a dying person compassionately practicing the healing of another is unforgettable. No doubt it's healing for the spirit and mind of the sick person doing the practice, and it probably benefits the person the Compassionate Breathing is directed to.

Through compassion we give and we heal. Like thousands and thousands of people before you, you can do this practice. It's within your natural capability. Healing is basic to your life, basic to your life force. You are the healer who makes more than 50,000 different biochemicals to dissolve potentially toxic substances that enter your body. You are the life force that empowers your immune system. If you look into it, you may have unlimited healing energy. This is a gift you have to offer. You are being asked to use this gift, for your sake and for the sake of others. The practice can be applied to any disease condition.

The Essential Practice

THE PRACTICE IS THIS: letting go of the concept that you are suffering a disease, dropping that as completely as possible to practice healing, forgetting yourself, with relief, you turn your focus to another person suffering the same sickness, or anyone suffering as much as you. You forget yourself and open your heart to the suffering person. You let go of who you think you are and what you think your body is.

Spontaneously you just follow your breath. Whatever your body is it's just breathing naturally in and out. Opening yourself completely to the person who is suffering, on the in-breath you take in, you energetically breathe in, all the sickness and suffering of the other person, wherever they are. Effortlessly, with empathy, you take the energy of their suffering into yourself with your inhale, and you see that energy naturally dissolve into light in your body. Effortlessly you breathe out into that person all the energy they need to heal. You are born to do this. You are universal. You can and should do this. What you inhale dissolves in light in you. You envision that the energy you send out, radiate out, intend out, *heals* and *frees* the other of sickness and suffering.

In your intention to heal another person you activate healing in yourself. That is the essence of the magic. That is the practicality of the method. If you do it sincerely you can and will experience how you can help others and heal yourself in the process.

In Compassionate Breathing we breathe in, taking in the energy of sickness and suffering—that of others or our own. We specifically take it into our light nature, into multidimensional live light of our own mind-body. We do not intentionally dissolve the energy of sickness into our light—this is an important point. We see that what we take in naturally dissolves into light in our body; we simply let it happen. We see that it is in our multidimensional nature that we cannot get sick, or psychologically disturbed, by compassionately taking on sickness and suffering, that we are made to experience the energy of others' illness naturally dissolving into light in us.

One can do this practice for oneself, seeing one's whole life and practicing compassion with this method, or for another. One can practice for oneself before practicing for another. One can practice for oneself and another at once. One can practice for several people at once. The power of this practice cannot be overestimated.

We can and should be fearless; that's a basis of any healing practice. It is in the nature of the energy that compassion takes in that it automatically dissolves in live light in our body. We effortlessly take in that energy, unlike "psychic surgery." It effortlessly, automatically dissolves into our light nature. Compassionate Breathing is not psychic surgery. We do not manipulate what we take in. We take it in energetically with unobstructed openness.

With this practice we can see, as tens of thousands of people have seen before us, that we are not "stuck with" our suffering, that it is our nature to let it go and to practice healing instead. In practicing the healing of others we can heal ourselves. The opportunity to express love, to express compassion, is healing for both oneself and for the one we express the compassion to. In that double reality is true magic. In an age when there are probably more psychological disturbances than ever, and more undiagnosed and wrongly diagnosed disease conditions than ever before, we have, from perennial wisdom, a distinguished, proven method to spontaneously free us from conditioned states and, at the same time, enable us to effectively practice the healing of others.

In one of Shakespeare's most memorable passages he says:

The quality of mercy is not strained,
It droppeth as the gentle rain from heaven
Upon the place beneath; it is twice bless'd;
It blesseth him that gives, and him that takes ...
(*Merchant of Venice*, act IV, scene 1)

Even on one's deathbed one can turn away from being caught up in oneself, turning freely to bless and heal others. With such a method it's relatively easy for a dying person to become a healer and a giver of blessings. Dying people can readily turn away from the conditioning of their life and enter the dynamic potential of the unconditioned state.

Compassionate Breathing is therefore a perfect hospice method, working with the inner awareness of the comatose and others near death. Breathing effortlessly, we inhale all the sickness and suffering of that person's life, taking it all in as if it were our own. It dissolves into light within, and we breathe out love and wisdom into the dying person. We bless that person and we are blessed by that person as we take in their suffering as blessing. Then the practice of Compassionate Breathing is genius, helping dying people heal into death.

Reversal of Suffering

MEDIGRACE HAS DEVELOPED a method of Compassionate Breathing called *Reversal of Suffering*. It's designed to assist anyone with the release and healing of any form of suffering—for oneself and for others.

THE METHOD

◆

Reversal of Suffering

Introduction

It's traditionally best to start by doing the practice for yourself.
Spontaneously sensing your whole life at once, shifting into a
    new dimension,
enter your timeless, nonlocal nature, and see your life
from your birth all the way through to the possible causes of
    your death.
Seeing this as only you can, and as you will know it,
experience inevitable compassion for yourself and your life.
Both because of all the suffering in the world
and because of many difficulties you probably have had,
open your heart to your self.
On your in-breath, without contriving your breath,
you breathe in all the sickness and suffering of your life.
Take it to heart.
See that it naturally dissolves into live light in you.
Then, effortlessly,
breathe out into yourself all the energy you need to heal all the
    wounds life tends to experience; all that you may ever have.
See that what you take in energetically dissolves into living light
    in you.
Effortlessly breathe out into yourself all the energy needed to
    heal all of your life.
Many, many people have healed themselves with this practice.
The more you do the practice, the better the quality of your effort
and the more alive the intention, the more effective it will be.
Then do the practice for another,
and then for more than one person at a time.

The instructions are traditional.
They have proved effective through the ages.
They are in increasing use in the medical establishment now.

Please practice this method of healing, for yourself and for the
world.

The Practice

You can do something for anyone who is suffering
physical and/or mental distress,
yourself or anyone else.
You can practice Compassionate Breathing.
It's best to start with yourself.

Shifting into your timeless awareness,
sense your whole life deeply.
See your whole life from your birth through the present moment,
and sense the rest of your life as it will be,
through the final causes of your death.
Sense your whole life with compassion.
Following the natural flow of your breath,
on your in-breath take in all the sickness and suffering of your
    life.
The energy of anguish and illness you take in
naturally dissolves into the light in your body,
and you effortlessly breathe out healing energy into your life.

Easily and completely, in the flow of your breath, all at once,
breathe in the oldest traumas of your life and the final challenges
    you'll face.
You take them into living light in you,
and as you breathe out, give out
all the grace and compassionate energy you can use.
Please do this now.
You were made to be the healer of your life.

Turning to another person,
someone you know well who has mental or physical torment, or
    both,
someone your heart easily turns to, someone close to you.
In the natural flow of your breath
you effortless breathe in, take in the disease, the torment, the
    crisis.
It dissolves in live light in you,
and you effortlessly breathe out, radiate out into that person
energies that can reverse and heal their suffering.
You see that happen.
You see the energy go where it should go
and do what it should do.
Please do that now.

You easily breathe in, take in
the energy of someone's suffering,
someone you know, wherever they are.
What you take in dissolves into light alive in you,
and you breathe out, intend out
energies that can reverse and heal their suffering.
Please do that now.

The longer you intend healing into yourself or into another
the more inevitable that healing will come.
Please practice that now.

You can shift from one person to another,
and you can practice Compassionate Breathing
for more than one person at a time.
Please do that now.
Breathe in, absorbing their anguish or sickness.
See that you can take it in
and it immediately dissolves into light in you;

and breathe out healing energy into those people,
sensing their different conditions and needs.
No matter how much healing they need
you have that much to give and more.
Please practice your healing ability now.

Turn to a hospital you know.
Imagine all its departments and services.
Imagine all the people coming there,
hoping for help with so many different conditions.
Sense the good intentions and limitations of the hospital.
Sense how much more healing the patients need.
Following the natural flow of your breath,
whether it is a short breath or a long one,
understand that we live in unified field.
Understand that the hospital is inside you.
Understand that you can breathe in, easily take in
all the sickness and suffering in the hospital.
Begin to know your unlimited nature.
Know your unlimited healing capability.
Practice the healing of everyone in the hospital at once.
Keep doing it until you see that you can.
Please do that now.

This is universal field medicine,
transpersonal medicine.
You go beyond yourself, beyond what you think you can do,
and you do it because at last it's time to experience that.
It is time to know your deep healing capability.
It's time to know how much healing you can do.
It's time to know how much healing needs to be done.
It's time to see that we touch the world more than we know.
It's time to practice healing touching all life.
Please do that now.

This is transpersonal medicine (Dossey 1993), universal field medicine. Because there is no separation of anyone or anything in the unified, universal field, you directly reach anyone in yourself, especially yourself. Just breathe in and take in the sickness and suffering of someone wherever they are, and breathe out all the energy the greatest healer could give. The practice can be done anywhere, anytime. We need only two things: the willingness to practice the healing of others by experiencing unlimited inherent healing energy in our systems, and the willingness to experience compassion, our natural ability to love, to do good.

Mother Teresa said it beautifully:

Loving as He loves,
Helping as He helps,
Giving as He gives,
Serving as He serves,
Rescuing as He rescues,
Being with Him twenty-four hours,
Touching Him in his distressing disguise.
(Sogyal 1994, 208)

Mother Teresa, like the Buddhist saints, *was* compassionate medicine.

References

Dossey, Larry. *Healing Words: The Power of Prayer and the Practice of Medicine.* New York: HarperCollins, 1993.
———. *Reinventing Medicine.* New York: HarperCollins, 1999.
Sogyal Rinpoche. *The Tibetan Book of Living and Dying.* New York: HarperCollins, 1994.

CHAPTER 11

Applications
Around Childbirth

THOUGH VARIOUS DISCIPLINES within the broad field of medicine have become interested in mind-body and energy medicine, the field of obstetrics, conceivably the most important field of medicine, is at once most in need of change and most resistant to change. But the world does change, in its steady, dynamic movement, and the widespread interest in the new areas of medicine has encouraged the development and presentation of new childbirth methods.

When Dr. Grantly Dick-Read (1944) and Dr. Fernand Lamaze (1958) developed their natural childbirth programs, they both had a sincere interest in the potential of mind-body methodology, but meditation science had not yet emerged as a major option of method and wisdom in the West. In the 1990s meditation science emerged as a mature and ready source of method and wisdom capable of revolutionizing the embattled field of obstetrics, able to slowly and powerfully enter that field to irreversibly change obstetric practices forever. The forces of history that seemed to doom life in the Cold War era gave life an opportunity to utilize a higher order of methodology in the support of childbirth as we entered the new millennium, methodology capable of raising the evolutionary quality of the species.

There was another powerful force energizing the potential of methodology change in childbirth, the force of the natural genius of womankind, repressed for hundreds of years, wanting to return to empowerment in the childbirth process in which womankind had been disempowered for so long.

Now, in the new millennium, the same forces of history have given us a remarkable opportunity to transform the process of childbirth. As the paradigm shifts and more and more people engage in the shifting of the childbirth paradigm, we are grateful that history is giving us a chance to raise the level of childbirth at this time. Life is ours to live while we have it, and we have the potential to evolve the paradigm right now.

What is the new childbirth methodology now so wonderfully available? It is both deep and multidimensional. We divide it into three areas:

- reclining meditation, based on progressive neuromuscular release, with the potential to heal the nervous system, and to raise the level of vitality and potential of function

- energy body–based sitting meditation, which presents a new vision of the body and its potential function as it helps to release any fear associated with childbirth

- transformative healing practice, which offers women the potential to regain their inherent healing powers

The Calm Birth program, developed by MediGrace in the 1990s, has been at work in the medical establishment since 1998. It offers practices that address all three areas, practices that have been gaining increasing support from childbirth professionals. The Calm Birth method has been refined through application for eight years in all three categories. The practices for prenatal care are fully presented in the book *Calm Birth: New Method for Conscious Childbirth* (Newman 2005), and on a CD audio-guide (CB3, via the Calm Birth website: www.CalmBirth.org). In this book we have chosen to present the Calm Birth postnatal care practices, previously unpublished:

- *Calm Mother*
- *Sitting into Energy Body*
- *Calm Parents, Calm Child*
- *Practice of Healing*

Calm Mother

JACOBSON'S GROUNDBREAKING WORK in neuromuscular release (1938) was further advanced in the medicine/meditation program at the University of Massachusetts Medical Center in 1979. The individual practicing one of Jacobson's Progressive Relaxation (PR) methods may have had trouble maintaining focus, and yet, remarkably, Jacobson's PR self-care methods were consistently effective. At UMMC, the application of mindfulness meditation to the practice of moment-by-moment neuromuscular release made the practice more efficient. Instead of randomly losing attention, the genius of mindfulness meditation enabled the individual to maintain the energy of attention on the practice, resulting necessarily in a more effective practice of release, with a greater potential for healing the nervous system.

The Calm Birth program utilizes mindfulness-based progressive neuromuscular release, with more dimension and potential in the practice, to help bring childbirth-related practices into a new domain of health. The pressures of life in the Age of Anxiety call for both prenatal and postnatal care methods of a higher order, to maintain and advance the empowerment of the woman, to heal her nerves of any birth-related stresses or disturbances, and to help the child access a higher level of development.

In the reclining meditation practice of *Calm Mother,* efficient neuromuscular release is applied to the aftermath of a labor and delivery process still too-often dominated by medical interventions such as drugs, anesthesia, and surgery—all of which impair nervous system function. Healing the nervous system after birth is as important as the use of neuromuscular release in preparation for birth. And just as both maternal and fetal nervous systems benefit from this healing practice in preparation for birth, both maternal and infant nervous systems benefit from *Calm Mother* in postnatal care. The child picks up benefits through sympathetic resonance, and, via lactation and breast-feeding, absorbs corresponding hormonal benefits, enhancing immune function and general systems function.

Another dimension of MediGrace's progressive neuromuscular release in postnatal care is engagement with physical light on a cellular level. This builds vitality needed for the demands of extensive postnatal responsibilities, emotions, and disordered sleep. The postnatal experience of physical inner light enhances the woman's sense of her body, facilitating healthy self-respect and continued empowerment.

The Method

Calm Mother

Following is a version of the audio-guide transmission of the method. You can obtain the audio-guide and experience the method through audio-guidance.

Introduction

This practice is done lying down.
It's a proven method to heal the nervous system.
It can free your nerves from labor and birth stress still in you.
This practice also brings you vital internal energy.
It can be a resource for years to come.
It's good for healing and regaining inner strength.
You progressively gain life force
and release disturbance and stress.

In this practice you go through your whole body,
progressively relaxing more and more.
You can have complete release and new energy.
The energy is essential for healing
and it brings calm.

Find yourself a comfortable place to lie down.
You can lie down on your bed.
But if you lie on blankets on a rug,
or on a yoga mat and a blanket,
you'll probably be more alert and gain more from the practice.
You'll be able to have moment by moment conscious release.
It's important to be comfortable and warm.
The effects are immediate
and they increase over time.
The most benefits come from daily practice.
Lie down mindfully.
Understand that you're not lying down to take a nap.
Please avoid falling asleep.
Keep your eyes open and softly focused.
This practice asks you to sense and enter
many dimensions of life in you,

so that you can realize more and more life.

It's good to close your eyes, from time to time,
but if you keep your eyes closed too much
you may tend to fall asleep.

The Practice

To begin, take a deep breath,
and then exhale easily.

Feel life energy working throughout your body.
Take another deep breath, deep into life,
and breathe out release, for greater function.

As if you're doing it for the first time
come into your whole body of life.
Feel the trillions of cells and the energy flows.
Let your self feel the dynamic of all your systems.

There's so much life in you it's inconceivable,
ten trillion living cells,
all working together as life force.

When you feel your whole body directly
you feel its unlimited life.
Keep feeling the sensation of all the pulsing currents,
the billionfold electric body process.
Feel all the life going on in you at once.
Feel your self start to become all alive.

As you become aware of life itself in you,
relax into it.
If there's any discomfort or pain

let go of that. Let it unfold.
Let it flow out.
See how you tend to hold onto tension.
See how you can let it all go.

Let go of any stress or disturbance.
You're going to take this time to relax deeply,
all the way through, slowly but surely.

Soon you'll go part by part through your body,
releasing the tension, feeling your energy increase.
You'll release the muscle tension on your nerves.
For the sake of your nervous system
you need to release your muscular tension.
You do that with internal life support,
from your feet to the crown of your head.

Starting with the toes of your feet,
feel all the life in your toes.
It's surprising how alive they are.
Feel their energy channels.
Feel the life in their bones.
Feel the channels and bones together in your feet.
Feel all their muscles and nerves.
Feel how it all works together.
Relax the muscles, tendons, and nerves.
Feel in your feet the service they've been giving you all these
    years.
Let them open into the full current of life.
Relax your feet into their open and ready state.
Feel how this benefits your arteries and nerves.

Bring your attention from your feet
up through your ankles, into your calves.

Feel all the energy flowing through them,
to and from all parts of your body.
Feel the life in the interconnection.
Find any tight muscles or tendons in your calves.
Relax the flesh and bone into its softness,
pliant and able.

Feel the goodness of the electrical flow,
the goodness of the blood flow,
the connection with the billionfold flows in your body.
Feel how deeply it's all connected.
Feel the deep dimensions of your life.
Feel the total connection everywhere in you now.

Come up from your calves into your knees.
Feel the life force in your knees.
This is a good way to meditate,
with moment by moment attention to the living systems in your
    body,
releasing stress on your nerves.
You gain force as you release,
freeing yourself into greater function.

Come up into your thighs.
Feel how they support your body.
Feel all their muscles and nerves.
Release all that needs to be released.
Optimize the aliveness of your flesh and bone.

Now bring your attention up into your hips.
Feel the muscles, nerves, and blood flow throughout your hips
    and buttocks.
Notice any unnecessary tension.
Please soften it. Rest it all.

Release tensions and let your nerves come into greater function.
Unlock and unblock, taking care of your own needs,
to have more to give to your child and family.
Let go of any restrictions.
Come into the basis of new life.

Bring your attention into your belly.
Sense if you hold any anxiety there.
Please breathe into your belly.
You can let go of anxiety.
You can relax and enter greater life.
Now is the time to help your self heal from any birth-related
    surgery or disturbance.
You can free yourself now.
Come into greater function.

Feel your womb and all your inner female organs.
If there's any energy of disturbance there
you can heal it now. Let that release.
Feel all the fine tissue there, and the nerves.
Breathe deeply into your womb,
exhaling easily, releasing whatever needs to be released.
Bless and heal whatever needs to be healed.
Feel all the forces of life blessing and sustaining you.
Direct blessing and sustenance to your female organs.
Whether you had a natural or a medicated birth
feel that your organs are sacred.
The experience of the sacred is what you need,
and it is in you, waiting.

Place your hands lightly on your belly.
Touch your sense of the sacred with sacred hands.
Feel the life force in your arms and hands.
Feel your healing ability in your hands.

Feel how much life you have to give to your child.
Feel how much care and grace you have to give.
Feel whole and healed in your self as the source of life.
Rest in your radiance and power.

Now bring your attention into your spine.
Feel the vertical force that carries your body.
Let your spine release and extend.
See the bones align.

Now feel your muscles throughout your rib cage and chest.
Release any tension there.
Let the muscles in your chest be free.
Feel your breasts alive with milk.
Feel the nourishment and gift in your milk.

Now feel the power of your heart.
Breathe love directly from your heart into your milk.
Feel your heart beating for you and your child.
Feel it sustain you.
Feel it beat for all you love.
Pulse in union with all you love.

Bring your attention to your upper back, shoulders, and neck.
Stress and tension tend to be held there.
Breathe into that area and relax any accumulated tension.

Take your time.

Let the tension melt away.
Let your self be naturally free of any stress.

Bring your attention into your face.
Feel your jaw and your mouth.

Let your lower face relax.
Feel all the muscles around your mouth,
forming your conscious and unconscious expression.
Let all your expression there release.
Feel your mouth become free.

Bring your attention up to your eyes.
Feel all the muscles around them,
holding conscious and unconscious expression of your life.
Relax all that completely. Let it go.
Let your face become completely free.
Feel your awareness become free.

Feel the depth of your calm.
Resting in soft open eyes
your energized body brims with life.
After giving birth you are reborn.
You have much more life to give.
You have much more life to receive.
You have unlimited reserves.

As you finish the practice and start to arise,
lift your self completely alive.
Prepare to give and receive life
as you move.

Sitting into Energy Body

I N THE 1990s an advanced form of mindfulness meditation, energy body–based transformative breathing, emerged as a method for both prenatal care and postnatal care. Energy body–based transformative breathing is called *Womb Breathing* in prenatal care. In postnatal care it is called *Sitting into Energy Body.*

If a woman has used *Womb Breathing* in prenatal care she will probably be interested in the postnatal care application of that method. If a woman has not used *Womb Breathing* in prenatal care, she may be interested in *Sitting into Energy Body* to give her a new potential of empowerment and capability in postnatal care and beyond.

Sitting into Energy Body is a sitting meditation based on this book's model of human anatomy, in which the physical body and the energy body are inseparable. It draws on the *Vajrayana* Buddhism of Tibet, in which one breathes energy from the air for greater function. In postnatal care, where so many women carry disempowerment from the childbirth process, consciously, unconsciously, or both, a practice like *Sitting into Energy Body*, with a transformative sense of body and breathing, is empowering.

Visualization

There are two major aspects of visualization in this practice: what breathes and what is breathed. Because both require a revolutionary sense of the function of the human body and the life-field in which the body lives, both need to be appropriately described. Concerning what breathes, for most people it is a revelation that our bodies were made to breathe energy as well as oxygen from the air for the full potential of human function. As well as breathing oxygen into the lungs, at the same time we are made to breathe energy from the air into a soft, luminous breathing feature in the navel center of our radiant energy body, from which our dynamic vertical series of power centers *(chakras)* arises. The body of full human function has millions of energy channels, but for the practice of *Sitting into Energy Body* we visualize just the CEC, with its *chakras,* and the soft, radiant Life Vase from which it rises.

With respect to what is breathed, we visualize that what we call *air* is a field alive with universal energy. In it is vital energy fundamental to everything alive. In some meditation science traditions it's called universal *chi;* in others, universal *prana.*

It's the fundamental or essential energy of all living things, and human beings are made to breathe it. We've been breathing it in and out all our lives without using it. In order to breathe it we sense it and breathe it in, intending it down into the Life Vase. When we breathe it and intend it down into the Vase we feel it go into the Vase. We bring ourselves into more complete function this way. In postnatal care we bring ourselves into a body of new potential and capability. We realize inherent dimensions of our body as if for the first time, when they are greatly needed. Especially if the woman is one of the more than 90 percent who did not experience full function of her womb while giving birth, due to drugs or anesthesia, this practice can be one of empowerment for the womb after birth.

THE METHOD

Sitting into Energy Body

Following is a version of the audio-guide transmission of the method. You can obtain the audio-guide and experience the method through audio-guidance.

Introduction

By sitting to calm and go deep
you can transform breathing and mind.
You can practice energy body after giving birth.
You can breathe energy into your energy body.

After giving birth you can practice power.
You can breathe energy into your Vase of Life.
In the beginning it's best to do this sitting practice
with audio-guidance.
The audio-guide practice takes twenty minutes.
Please use the CD as a basis of daily practice.
Each time the instructions become clearer.
Even when you know the instructions by heart
it's still good to practice at least twenty minutes,
and it's best to practice early in the day.

You sit to develop power to start the day.
You sit to come alive with energy.
You sit to reach deep reserves and start the day with joy.
Then throughout the day it's best to sit down
and regain the practice, for a few minutes each time.
If you sit and stop the world,
stopping to breathe energy into your energy body,
your body will take up the practice instinctively.
More and more the practice will come to you from the inside.
The more you do the practice,
the more you'll realize your energy body as your potential.

So sit down into your body to shift into your strength.
Sit to calm and breathe in a deeper way.
Sit on a cushion on the floor

or sit in a chair, balanced and at ease.
Effortlessly keep your spine upright,
so that it naturally lifts.
Feel your balance and stability.
Now visualize your body in a deeper way.

See that inside your body is a body of energy channels.

See the energy body that meditation science has used for
    centuries,
helping people come into their power and full development.

See the vertical series of energy power centers,
from the crown of your head down into your navel.

This is the central energy channel, the wisdom channel.

At the bottom of the central energy channel, in its navel center,
is the Vase of Life,
a soft, luminous breathing Vase from which the central channel
    rises.
It's there for you to bring energy up into your energy body.

You breathe energy from the air into the Vase.
From the Vase the energy feeds up into the central energy
    channel,
to bring the higher systems of your body to life.

Many, many people have done this practice,
for centuries, breathing energy from the air into the Vase of Life,
to come alive with greater function, greater ability.
Please sit and breathe this way.
Sense the vital energy in the air.
It's always been there.

It's been called *prana*, or *chi*.
It's the universal energy that makes everything alive.

The *prana*, the *chi*, is the basis of your life.
You were born to breathe this vital energy in the air.
That same energy is the basis of your body.

The Practice

Begin by sensing the *chi* in the air,
sense that you were born to breathe it into the Vase,
the soft, radiant Vase at the base of your central channel.
All your life you've been breathing this vital energy without
    using it.
Now breathe it in
and intend it down into the Vase.
When you do you'll feel it go into the Vase.
Please breathe life-giving energy into the Vase of Life.

Sense your body deeply.
Feel life sensation throughout your body.
Feel and see the breathing Vase in your navel center,
a soft energy Vase within your physical body.
Know that you were made to breathe vital energy to be more
    alive.

Breathe in the vital energy from the air to be more alive.
Feel that you're breathing life energy down near your womb.
Feel how you're doing this to empower your womb.
Breathe energy into the Life Vase near your womb.

As you sit and breathe in this deeper way,
this healthier way,
breathing and intending vital energy down into the Vase,

your mind tends to distract you.
Instead of breathing vital energy for greater function
you may find yourself lost in thought,
thinking about something that happened,
or something that's going to happen.
You may be distracted.

Then something in you wants to wake up.
Something in you, free of your mind,
wakes you up and brings you back.

Come back to energy breathing.
Come back to breathing with your energy body.
Breathe energy into the Vase of Life.
Empower yourself after giving birth.
Breathe energy with awareness to become more alive.

Sense the universal field of life.
Sense the universal energy field.
Sense the *prana,* the *chi* of that field,
the field that gives you life.
Sense the life-giving field all around you and in you.
Sense that the life-field is breathable.
Sense that you can breathe its energy.
This energy is given to you to use.
You can breathe it and use your body in a new way.
You can live in a greater way after giving birth.
You can have more energy to serve life.

You're doing what is right for you to do.
Breathe in a greater way.
Breathe full oxygen and vital energy.
You'll have more life to give to life.
Your mind may interfere,

but your awareness is free of your mind.
Breathe with awareness, free of your mind.
You'll start to see what your mind is.
You've been giving your power to your mind all your life.
This is the time for revolution.
Shift your power from your mind to your awareness.
Breathe vital energy with awareness.

Your mind may try to take you away.
The more you practice breathing life energy with awareness,
the more awareness you have,
the more you can breathe in a greater way.
Breathe life into your Vase and have more life to give,
to your child, to your family, to the world.
Breathe in the only revolution.
Breathe to shift power into greater life.

Sometimes you'll wake up in the morning breathing this way.
You'll sit down into the calm that comes with breathing this way.
You'll sit down into quiet energy.
In that quiet is the stillness of a higher order.
Breathe into energy body for greater life.

You can go to sleep this way.
Sit and calm into greater function.
Establish breathing into the Vase.
Raise the intention to breathe vital energy in your sleep.
Your unconscious mind can breathe energy in your sleep.
It can give you a deeper kind of rest.
You can rest relaxing into greater function.
Then you'll awake into a different kind of life.

Breathe into a different kind of life.
Practice revolution into grace.

Shift your attention from your mind to your awareness.
Practice breathing life-giving energy in the air.
Practice breathing vital energy to have more life to give.
Receive the life-giving energy field that makes the world alive.
Use the energy you were born to use.

Breathe life into yourself
and your child will gain life.
Your child will gain awareness and energy
in sympathetic resonance with you.
Other children or family will gain energy in sympathetic
    resonance with you.
Your child, your children, will pick up your energy and calm.
Please do this practice for yourself and others.
Please do this practice to give life to life.
Please continue breathing into the Vase.

Calm Parents, Calm Child

THIS IS A NEW MEDITATION PRACTICE designed to doubly benefit the newborn child. It brings the dual meditation of mother and father into the child in the same way at the same time.

Mother and father sit on opposite sides of the child while it sleeps. They let the child teach them to breathe. Then they let the child teach them to:

- heal into calm
- breathe into new life
- breathe into new world
- sense many dimensions of the child's life
- sense the greatness of life
- breathe into the source of that life
- breathe into the greatness of life
- send and receive the blessing of life
- feel the power of life
- accept life from the child
- feel sustained by the life of the child

For father, mother, and child, and for all mothers—all parents—and children, a deeper, calmer postpartum experience becomes possible because one is doing these practices. The morphic field of parenting is affected every moment that one mother or father stops and breathes and remembers the true nature of being and of relationship, knowing peace, for themselves and their child.

THE METHOD

Calm Parents, Calm Child

Following is a version of the audio-guide transmission of the method. You can obtain the audio-guide and experience the method through audio-guidance.

Introduction

Mother and father do this meditation with your baby,
while the child sleeps.
Sit in chairs, or on cushions on the floor,
as near as possible to the child.

The Practice

Let yourselves settle down.
Bring your breathing down.
Breathe with your bellies.
Breathe the way the baby breathes.

Be like the child.
Breathe in peace.

Keep your bodies upright and balanced.
Sit still, and come to rest.

Breathe with the baby.
Let your minds quiet.
Become still with the child.
Let motion cease.
Let your minds calm.

Breathe with the babe.
Let the child teach you to breathe.
Sense the child's inner awareness.
Let the three of you rest in union.
Come into living presence.
Breathe in living presence....

Breathe with new life in the child.
Breathe with new world in new life.

When your mind starts to talk,
shift into open awareness.
Bring your breathing down.
Find stillness in the child.
Sense many dimensions in the child.
Sense the greatness in all that life.
Breathe into cohesion with that.
Breathe into the source of life.
Breathe into the greatness of life.

Sense the blessing of life.
Receive the blessing of life.
Give the blessing of life.

Feel life itself pulsing in you.
Feel life itself pulsing in you three.
Feel the calm that heals.
Breathe calm.
Breathe grace,
one with the child.

Feel the power of life.
Feel sustained by life.
Feel sustained by the child.
Feel blessed by the child.
Be blessed by the babe.

Accept life from the child.
Give calm to each other.
Receive grace this way.
Give grace this way.

Breathe with the child.
Open to life.
Open to receive.
Open to give.
In open awareness
be blessed by the child.

Receive calm.
Rest in grace.
Give into peace.

Give the child peace.
Give each other peace.
Give the world peace.

Breathe into life.

Breathe life into life.

When you both arise
continue to breathe with the child.

Your teacher is here.
Your teacher is here.

Practice of Healing

G*iving and Receiving* is an application of Transformative Compassionate Breathing for childbirth. Applied to the postpartum experience, MediGrace calls it *Practice of Healing*. This practice gives the new mother a method for healing through breathing and seeing. The practice is used to reverse any adverse condition in the woman or in the child. *Practice of Healing* can bring healing and grace into motherhood.

The process is elegantly simple. Naturally coming into her breathing at any moment, following the natural flow of the breath, the new mother breathes in the energy of any adverse condition in herself or in her child. That energy instantly dissolves into light in her, and she breathes out healing energies into herself and her child, practicing energy medicine.

Practiced for oneself, *Practice of Healing* is a transformative self-healing practice. Practiced for another, it's doubly healing (see Chapter Ten).

The meditation is inseparable from the genius of the human life force. It's the great doctor in the immune system, and more. Seeing herself as only she knows herself, seeing her whole life, from birth to death—and only she can know it—she breathes in, takes in, takes on all the sickness and pain of her life; it dissolves into the light in her body, and then she breathes out into herself all the compassion and healing she could ever need. She takes in all the pain and stress of her life, and openheartedly breathes into herself that which heals her life. The practice is equally effective in calming and healing her child.

THE METHOD

Practice of Healing

Following is a version of the audio-guide transmission of the method. You can obtain the audio-guide and experience the method through audio-guidance.

Introduction

After giving birth
it's empowering to practice healing.
There's a famous practice
used for centuries
for healing and empowerment.

It's a practice of healing
using Compassionate Breathing.

It's very powerful.
It has transformed many people.
It's always good for women
to practice their innate ability to heal others.

If a woman has given birth with surgery or drugs,
she can heal herself and her child of the side effects
and she can heal herself of any surgical wound.
Though medical birth heals by itself she can heal it faster.

If a woman had a natural childbirth
she has used deep resources.
It's good for her to practice Compassionate Breathing.

The more you practice healing yourself and your child
the more profound your health and the child's health will be.
The more you practice healing others
the stronger your inherent healing genius will be.
The more you practice Compassionate Breathing,
and the more you teach the practice to others,
the more you'll help other women develop inner resource.

The Practice

You begin by practicing healing for yourself.
You sense your whole life,
all the way from your birth on into your present and future life.
Sensing that most people have some disturbance or trauma in
    being born,
and you probably did,
follow the natural flow of your breath.

On the in-breath breathe in the energy of any disturbance or
    harm
that may remain from your own birth.
See that energy naturally dissolve into light in your body.
Breathe out into your birth
the healing energy it may need.

This practice is far-reaching.
You can easily breathe back into your birth.

Breathe in any energy from your birth that may need to be
    cleared.
See it dissolve into natural light in you.
Breathe out into yourself compassionate energy
that can completely heal your birth.

It's time to heal with the breath.
Please do that now. . . .

Now turn your attention to all of your life.
Remember whatever sickness and suffering you had.
Some of the energy of that may have stayed in your mind.

On your in-breath effortlessly take that in.
See that what you take in dissolves in light in your body,
and you breathe out into yourself compassionate energy
that can heal whatever remains to be healed.
It's time to be free of the past.
It's time to be healed and empowered with your breath.
Please complete your healing and empower yourself now....

Turning to the recent birth of your child,
if it was a medical birth
you can heal side effects that can linger from that.
If it was a natural birth
take this time to heal any suffering that may have come up.
On your in-breath take in anything at all that can and should be
    healed,
in you and in your child.
It's time to dissolve that into light in you.
Easily breathe out into yourself and your child
all the healing energy you both may need.
You can complete the birth now.
You can heal with Compassionate Breathing.
Please do that now....

Turning your attention completely to your baby
for a few breaths breathe your energy into and out of the child,
sensing your deep ability to help.
There may be disturbances in the child
that were experienced while in the womb.
There may be disturbances in the child
from a previous life.

Sensing your far-reaching ability with this practice
as you breathe in take out of the child
and into yourself any disturbance or harm

that remains in your child from the past, including the time in
   your womb.
The miracle is that you cannot take on that suffering or
   disturbance
if you compassionately breathe it in.
It must dissolve into live light in your body,
light essential to your nature.
You're able to take in disturbance from your child
and see it naturally dissolve into your inner light.
You're able to breathe out into the child
energy vital for its body and mind.
You can do this if you try.
Please do this now. . . .

Turning to other people around you,
people important to you and your child,
focus on them one by one.
Practice your natural healing ability.
Effortlessly following the flow of your breath,
feeling your connection with someone close to you, wherever
   they are,
inhale into yourself the energy of any suffering or disturbance
   they may have.
See that what you take in dissolves into light in your body,
and lovingly breathe out into that person healing energy they
   may need.
Please practice healing now. . . .

Turn to someone else that you know,
someone who could be helped more than they know.
Wherever they are you reach them immediately in yourself.
As you breathe in take in the energy of any harm or health
   challenge they may have.
See that you can take into yourself that which can make them free.

See that what you take in dissolves into light in your cells,
and effortlessly send out into that person energy they need to
    heal and be free.
Give out your healing energy bountifully.
As you send it out to someone in the world
extra energy flows forward beyond them,
flowing out into the universe, accomplishing secret healings.
Please practice your ability to heal.
Please practice Compassionate Breathing now....

Throughout the course of the day,
while taking care of yourself and your child,
please practice Compassionate Breathing.

The more you practice healing for yourself and your child
the more whole and free you both will be.

The more you practice the healing of others,
the more you will empower yourself.

The more you benefit others in the world
the more you can make this a better world.

Please do this practice of healing often.
    As with all the MediGrace methods, this one can be practiced
in the transpersonal domain. It can be practiced for all the women
in the world suffering postpartum distress. If a woman practices
these methods in her universal nature, her transpersonal nature,
she can affect the greater field of life. Awareness of our transpersonal nature, our unlimited connection with life, and awareness of
our unlimited power of intention, make these methods appropriate for an emerging new era of healing.

References

Dick-Read, Grantly. *Childbirth Without Fear*. New York: Simon & Schuster, 1944.

Jacobson, Edmund. *Progressive Relaxation*. Chicago: University of Chicago Press, 1938.

Lamaze, Fernand. *Painless Childbirth*. New York: Simon & Schuster, 1958.

Newman, Robert. *Calm Birth: New Method for Conscious Childbirth*. Berkeley, CA: North Atlantic Books, 2005.

CHAPTER 12

Healing the Present
by Healing the Past

O VER THE PAST CENTURY, the fields of psychology, psychiatry, psychotherapy, and counseling have been evolving in response to the emotional and mental disturbances of life in Western culture. These fields have advanced our understanding of the nature of mind and the relationship between mind and body. They have also all but eliminated the inhumane treatment of mentally disturbed and challenged people from the cultural norm. These fields have also provided much-needed relief for thousands of people suffering from chemical imbalances in the mind-body system.

They have not always been successful, however, in assisting the essentially healthy person who seeks to move on from a traumatic or distressing situation and establish a new norm. In fact, the use of medications and the tendency to focus on the past have been seen by many health professionals as well as the general public as undermining the health of the mind-body for those people whose needs are developmental rather than remedial.

Outside of Western culture, such needs are typically met with methods designed to facilitate shifts in consciousness. In some cultures experiences that Western psychology might call "schizophrenic" or "psychotic" are understood to be stages in a developmental process. As anthropologist Gregory Bateson put it, "schizophrenia is a necessary stage on the spiritual path" (1972).

Thus far, we've explored a number of meditative processes that result in shifts of consciousness and facilitate healing processes. Each of them is designed to shift the practitioner's mind-body system from the limitations of normal mental/cognitive processes into a state of awareness that is free of such limitations.

One of those limitations is the idea of time.

In the world of quantum physics, the past and future are simply ideas and all that exists is this moment, now. Eckhart Tolle, in his remarkable story, *The Power of Now* (1999), makes it clear that when we can live without concern for the past or the future, the world is a light-filled space, with all that we need for this moment. It's only when we start to be upset about some past event or concerned about some future event that life gets unpleasant.

So, if we want to live fully in the energy of the present, we must release whatever is causing us to bring the past or future into this moment. Whatever thoughts or ideas we have about who we are that come from the past are probably no longer valid, and so we can let go of them and step into the infinite, boundless potentiality of this moment, now.

In shamanic traditions, this process is called "soul retrieval." Part of us, part of the fields of energy that we are, is still caught up in some event or relationship from the past. We need to retrieve that part of us and restore our sense of wholeness—releasing the memory and the emotions associated with it, in the process. The shaman facilitates that process, helping people see where we have left "a part of ourselves" and helping them return to their innate wholeness and completeness.

Methods for Transforming the Past

A S WE CONSIDER THE REALITY that the past does not exist in any physical sense, but exists only in our memories, then we open the door to the possibility of transforming those memories. Shamans

have understood this for millennia and New Thought practitioners have worked with the idea for more than a hundred and fifty
years. We offer here two practices: one from ancient tradition in
Tibetan Buddhism, and one that is derived from the principles and
practices of New Thought.

Sacred Fire

IN *Vajrayana* Buddhism there is a practice, handed down through the ages, that enables people to change the past, if they are willing to act for the benefit of all life. It is a sacred fire practice called *Riwo Sang Cho.* The practice takes about forty-five minutes to perform. It may be done by one person alone, or by two people, one of whom manages the fire. Or it may be done as a group practice. In that case the person most experienced with the practice makes the preparations and leads the ceremony and chanting. Everyone participating will know the meanings of the activity and each person will act to heal his or her own past karma and larger fields of karma, each person acting on behalf of all life while experiencing the additional power of the force field of the group. According to the visionary genius of this practice, everyone who has ever lived is still alive and accessible in an energetic field, in transpersonal dimensions, until they are freed from karmic consequences maintaining that field.

The fire *puja* can be an elaborate ritual, as described below, in which a sacred mixture called *sang* is offered in the fire, or it can be as simple as offering the same practice with a stick of incense. Some incense is made for that purpose. In either case the effectiveness of the practice depends on the power of one's intent, the ability to offer in the smoke intention to heal the past, on many levels. Essential to healing the past through this practice is the intention to see and access one's past negative karma and the negative karma of all sentient beings. This includes killing, causing many kinds of psychological harm, deception, stealing, and breaking vows. The practice may be done simultaneously to free one's own past and the species' past of negative karma, including healing personal and species-wide illnesses and disturbances that are the result of past negative actions.

THE METHOD

❦

Sacred Fire

Introduction

You can do the practice in your ordinary form, but it's more effective when done through accessing your sacred nature and full potential. The confidence of that vision is comparable with the confidence needed to make an infinite offering with the power of intent. The offering is made to fill vast space and reach the past unlimitedly, reaching all of the past of your present life and reaching into all of your past lives, and simultaneously doing that for all sentient beings. You can reach an unlimited number of lives. Beings that we have karmic debts with are waiting to be free of that. On another level all life is waiting to be freed of larger fields of negative karma, personal, cultural, historical, and planetary. According to what each individual may believe they need to free them of various past karmic consequences, they will see that in the light and smoke of the offering fire. The smoke is compassion. The offering gives liberating energy to all those you have unresolved karma with, in this and past lives, and all beings in the larger karmic fields. You see that they all receive what they think they need to free them through the power of your intention, and they actually receive what they really need for freedom on all levels. What they actually need is your ability to see that everyone is their inherent buddha-nature, all-knowing awareness, free of life and death.

Throughout the offering, periodically, for substantial periods, the mantra "OM AH HUNG" is recited, three brilliant seed syllables, aligned to empower body, speech, and mind. As you recite, you envision the smoke carrying "OM AH HUNG" as a liberating offering to all life throughout all time. What everyone receives is an energizing "OM AH HUNG." The OM is the energy of empowerment into sacred body, the purification of the body into buddha-body. The AH is the energy of the empowerment into sacred speech, the purification of ordinary speech into wisdom speech. The HUNG is the energy of empowerment into the all-knowing liberated mind of buddha-nature. All the beings you reach are forms of energetic imprints in a vast transpersonal field, and they receive your offering, healing and releasing obstructive energetic patterns. You liberate your past, present, and future and you liberate the past, present, and future of all. Essentially we're purifying our own energy bodies as the basis of purifying the world's countless energy bodies.

The Practice

For the elaborate practice, preparations are needed.

First there should be a dedicated fire-offering site, a place made for sacred ceremony. It should not be used for ordinary purposes. A consecrated mixture called *sang*, sacred offering, may be used. This offering mixture is prepared in a reverential process that can take hours to complete, and requires various ingredients, the most important of which are blessed substances. Among these may be grains of diamond, emerald, gold, or other precious or semiprecious substances consecrated by teachers of the lineage with the intention that they be offered in *Riwo Sang Cho* to release energies of the past that are obstructing the present and future of human life, for the sake of planetary progress. Consecrated herbs, silk of five colors, red, blue, green, gold, and white, cut into fine pieces, and five white substances, such as flour and sugar, are among the ingredients used. There is more that must be known to create the appropriate *sang*. You must learn all aspects of this important method from experienced practitioners.

The base of the fire should be made with clean wood and kindling. The primary substance to be burned, into which the *sang* mixture is added, is evergreen. Juniper is considered optimal, as it has been for the Native Americans. Cedar, spruce, and other evergreens are also good. Water is sprinkled onto the evergreen to assure that it will issue white, steamy smoke, rising from the flames, "a cloud of compassion." The *sang* mixture is added periodically, when the person directing the ceremony indicates to the person attending the fire. Those participating will see that as the *sang* burns it colors the light of the fire, making a sacred offering that invokes and works with the field of all time and all life. Beyond personal memory the past exists as a pattern in the vast transpersonal field that is accessible through this practice.

The practice is performed according to a ritual text in the *Vajrayana*. The text is chanted melodically. A ritual bell is used to add energetic emphasis at various times in the practice, especially when cutting the force of different aspects of the energy field of the past limiting life as we live it now. When the fire is well established, the person directing the practice and leading the chanting indicates to the person attending the fire to start adding the evergreen. Then the chanting begins.

First those present take two vows. The first vow is to attain realization to know life in its greatest dimensions. The second vow is to live and work for the benefit of all life.

Then the ritual language of the practice calls into the field of all life and all time, and describes what is being offered for the benefit of all life. For instance, the silk of five colors represents five kinds of human psychological poisons, anger, greed, envy, pride, and ignorance, transformed energetically in the fire into five kinds of corresponding enlightened energies. Various aspects of the energetic properties of the *sang* are offered as treasure to release karmic factors still active in the past that limit life in the present, and limit the potential of the future.

Finally, the ancient wisdom that is the basis of the practice reveals all the kinds of energetic karmic forces of the past that can be accessed and changed by this practice. Again and again those conditions are evoked, and again and again they are acted upon by the spiritual genius of the offering, until the process is complete.

During the practice, those participating look for signs, in the sky and in the environment. Sometimes there are extraordinary signs, such as a rainbow in a clear sky. But the signs vary due to the challenging conditions of human life.

After the recitation of the practice is completed, heart prayer is made into the field of all time and all life by those present. Some people act to heal their karma with their parents or others for whom they may have regrets based on unskillful actions that may have caused suffering. With this offering inordinate possibilities arise, especially if one is acting from the desire to benefit the greatest number of people possible.

After the practice is complete, people may use the fire to burn old photographs or letters, or anything else that one may dispose of in a sacred fire as an act to purify the past, and to free the present of past influences that may limit present life.

This practice suggests that tradition and community give us resources that are crucial to maintain and fully utilize if we are to access all our means to heal our lives and the world.

12 Steps to Freedom

ANYONE WHO HAS WRESTLED with the effects of alcoholism or drug addiction is familiar with the classic 12-step program of restoration. What they may not realize is that this program grew out of another 12-step program—one designed to transform ordinary Christians into powerful healers. This earlier program was designed originally by Mary Baker Eddy, who built the Christian Science Church around it at a time when women had little power and virtually no authority. It was modified by a remarkable scholar and teacher, Emma Curtis Hopkins, whose students built several denominations and the whole New Thought movement around it. One minister of that movement, Emmet Fox, helped to birth Alcoholics Anonymous, and his books, especially *Sermon on the Mount,* remain core texts for people who are working the program.

The method presented here includes elements of both the 12-step and Hopkins' programs, along with some ritual traditions from indigenous cultures. It's designed to help the individual get rid of old patterns of thought or belief—and the actions that result—that no longer contribute to a healthy, prosperous, enjoyable life.

The Method

12 *Steps to Freedom*

Introduction

This method is an internal process.

It's simple and relatively painless, and the first time may take several hours, or days (with breaks), to complete.

Ideally, it's done in privacy, where you can feel free to move around and make as much noise as you want.

All you need is something to write with, something to write on, a pillow or mattress, some warm, comfortable clothing, plenty of drinking water, and perhaps a box of matches.

The Practice

Step One. Awareness

Like the AA program, it's important to recognize that nothing happens until you realize something is not working. In systems thinking, this is called the "felt disequilibrium"—the recognition that something's out of whack and you don't want life to continue this way.

> Whenever your life is not "working," when you're not feeling joyful and satisfied, is a good time to stop and take stock. Stop what you've been doing and take some time alone. Consider: What is disturbing me? What am I experiencing and/or thinking that is not contributing to my well-being? What am I ready to let go of?

Step Two. Acceptance

Again, it's not possible to do something different until you've fully accepted that what has been is no longer okay.

> Calmly consider what you have discovered. Accept that it's no longer serving you and that you're ready for a change. Sit with it for a while. Relax in that acceptance. There's no need

to blame self or others, just an acceptance that what was going on before is no longer what you intend for your life.

Step Three. Acknowledgment

This one's a little tricky. Even though you've accepted that the situation you're in is not what you're willing to put up with anymore, you need to acknowledge that, somehow, this pattern has served you in the past. You wouldn't be who you are, with all the strengths and skills and abilities you have, without this in your life. So you bless it and acknowledge it for the contribution it has made in your life and world. Doing so, you dissolve some of the obstructions in your consciousness that are keeping you from experiencing a full, satisfying life.

Take time to remember the good times. This person, situation, activity, or thought is part of what made you who you are. Be aware of that for a while. Remember the times that it served you. *Feel* the appreciation that comes with those memories.

Then, be aware of the gratitude that you feel for those good times and for the contribution this has made in your life. If you don't feel it spontaneously, practice. Try saying, "Thank you for the good times; thank you for all the ways you've given me _____." Fill in the blank with a word or phrase, like "strength; understanding; the will to stand up for myself; skills and abilities I didn't have; opportunities to go places and meet people; a home; children." There are undoubtedly several things in your life that wouldn't be there without this person, situation, activity, or thought. As you practice, you will probably start feeling the appreciation.

Step Four. Expression

And, of course, as we appreciate something we're ready to let go of, all kinds of "buts" come up. This is normal and appropriate: it's how human beings move out of complacency to new levels of development. This is the first step in the process that is called, in New Thought, "negation" or "denial": when the situation, behavior, or thought is pushed out of the mind-body system. Often, this step happens in a therapist's office, which is fine and can be very effective. If that isn't possible or appropriate, however, it can be done at home—or in a safe, relatively isolated space where others won't be affected by the activities and sounds associated with it.

> The thoughts and feelings you've had about this have been stored in your whole mind-body: the muscles and nerves, as well as the brain. Depending on how long you've been uncomfortable and how far back in your lifetime this came in, they may be quite deep and intense.
>
> So this is not just a thought process; it's a whole-body activity. It's where the mattress or pillow come in—you may want to beat on them now and then as feelings come up in the body. It's also where writing it out may get hot and heavy— you probably have a lot of things you'd like to say to certain people. You may even want to shout a little, or even scream— it's okay: they can't hear you and you're not hurting anyone. You also may find that your arms or legs want to move, to shake, or to throw something—again, go ahead.
>
> It's all part of ex-pressing—pushing from—pushing away—this thing that you're ready to let go of.
>
> You'll know when you're done expressing when your body feels tired and kind of empty and you can't think of anything to say except maybe something like "and I know you really tried...."

Step Five. Release

The second stage in the "negation" step is releasing the situation or thought from the mind-body consciousness. This is an act of intention made visible. It's a way to tell the part that runs the mind-body system that this is no longer a part of the system and we're ready to live without it. It's what the shaman is doing when she or he sucks something out of someone's body and burns it. It's what the "burning bowl" rituals are for.

When you feel like there's nothing left to express, you get to pick up everything you've written and anything else that was part of your expression and let them go.

If you wrote your feelings down on paper, it's a good time to rip it all up into little shreds and maybe even burn it (hence the matches). If you didn't write anything, it's time to take all that energy you just spewed out into the room and pack it up into the Cosmic Garbage Bag. (Yes, we know you didn't really make a mess, and no, there isn't really a Cosmic Garbage Bag, but it's good for your psyche to pretend that you're really getting rid of this stuff—the unconscious mind doesn't know the difference between pretend and real activity!)

So burn the paper and watch the smoke dissipate in the heavens. Or take your imaginary yuk, put it in the imaginary bag, and put the imaginary bag into an imaginary rocket ship that's headed straight for the sun—it'll be transformed into healing light, there. Or take something that stands for all this outside and throw it as hard and as far into the ocean—or nearest river—as you can, and let it be purified by the water as it is washed away from you.

Then go take a shower and let the flowing water cleanse your physical body as its energy cleanses your energy body, washing any remnants of this issue down the drain.

Step Six. The Conversation

Having released, or "negated," the situation, it's time to transform our relationships with the people involved in this whole thing. In AA and other 12-step programs, this is the first part of the atonement step. And reconciling with the folks who've been injured through an addiction is an important thing to do in the recovery process.

However, we're not talking about the distress we've caused others, but the distress we're experiencing now as a result of things they've said or done in the past. And, as we stated previously, both science and mystical traditions agree that the only place the past exists is in our memory. Therefore, because the only place any of these people and their actions exist now is in our memory/imagination, then that's where we need to do the work. (If you don't believe this is true, ask a sibling or a friend to share his or her memories of a time that you remember from childhood and you'll see how different your experiences were—even of the same event!)

This process requires the most concentration. It's an imagery process in which the practitioner has a dialogue with the people who've helped bring him or her to this point in life. The skill is in sustaining the image—with as much detail and as many senses as possible—long enough to get through what needs to be said. If this is not a skill you've developed, you may want to precede this process with the Progressive Relaxation method described in Chapter Eight. It may take several shorter sessions, rather than one long one, to complete.

So get comfortable and, if it helps you to imagine more clearly, put a chair or that pillow in front of you.

Now imagine the person you have the most energy toward in this situation sitting there. See their face and eyes, how they wear their hair, how they hold their shoulders. See the colors they're wearing and what they have in their hands, if anything. Hear their voice speaking to you. Hear your own voice speaking to them, as you tell them everything you have to say—the good, the bad, and the ugly. Use all your senses to make this conversation as real as possible, so your subconscious mind knows that you've said all these things and it doesn't have to keep them in your surface mind, anymore.

Then, when you run out of steam, stop for a bit and listen. Hear what they have to say, if anything. You may be surprised by what you learn in this process.

You'll want to hold this conversation with everyone involved. You need to have them all hear everything you have to say, and you need to hear what they have to say to you. This may take a while and will require considerable concentration on your part, so don't give yourself too bad a time if you don't get through it all in one sitting.

Step Seven. Forgiveness

This is the second part of the atonement step in AA. Another way to think of this step is "giving-for-ness" (Miller 2005). In this step we are replacing the idea of hurt, shame, or pain with a new idea: wholeness, wellness, or simply "getting along."

This step usually happens as part of the imagined conversation, but it may happen in reverie or meditation following. It's complete when we know that we have released the people associated with this situation or thought, and we know that we are released as well. Whatever anger or blame or upset that we've held against them is released, and we are free. In the Christian tradition, this is the point of Baptism.

It may not seem possible that everyone involved in this can be forgiven, but, truly, it's the only way to get free. In fact, that's really what you've been doing in this imaginary conversation: in whatever words work for you, you've been saying, "I'm willing to let this go and move on from it, not carry it around anymore, and I hope you are too."

If you don't get a clear "yes" from your visualized companion at that point, you get to ask straight out: "Do you forgive me?" (If you're thinking this is crazy, yes, we know that you were the one who got hurt in this, but you're also the one who's been nursing a grudge for however long it's been.)

You're not done until you know that you've been forgiven. If all else fails, look up and ask your Higher Self, Jesus, Allah, or whatever you call God to do it for you—you can be sure of forgiveness there.

Note: If you can't tell whether you've completed this step or not, remember this line from *A Course in Miracles:* "You know you've forgiven someone when all you remember is the love between you."

Step Eight. Declaration

When we've fully forgiven, nothing exists except the moment: no past, no present, just the love. When we remember this, when we *feel* it, then all the potential of what Deepak Chopra calls "the field of infinite possibility" is available to us. This state is very close to the Buddhist state of *rigpa*—pure awareness. Here we are beginning what, in New Thought, is called "Affirming." We are declaring to the universe, and instructing our mind-body system, what we intend to experience. And, because our mind-bodies are "fields within fields" of energetic "wavicles" that align themselves in patterns of resonance with ideas, the ideas we choose have manifesting power—in our bodies and our world.

"When in the course ..." of achieving the State of Forgiveness, you arrive in a State of Grace. In this state is Power. In this Power, you get to ask for whatever you truly want—not just ask, but Claim!

But be careful—in this state, you *will* get what you wish for! So think of the highest possible good you can imagine coming out of this situation. Think of what would bring joy and well-being for all involved—especially you! And when you have a clear idea of it, say it. Out loud. And write it. In big, bold letters.

This is your next great step in life and you want to be very clear and strong as you take it.

Step Nine. Letting It Go

As we move through this process, the old situation seems less and less real. We are replacing it in our memories, and in our lives, with new images and new ideas. Our life moves forward in this new, transformed way without our having to pay attention to it—just as it always has. So we don't concern ourselves with it. It is done. Finished. Nothing.

Instead, we turn our attention to what is in front of us, the daily tasks of life, knowing that our intention is set and the energy of our mind-body system is working in harmony with the energy of the rest of the world to bring it to pass. This is the 12-step "Let go and let God." It's an act of trust, of faith, that the universe of which we are a part is, as Einstein said, "a friendly one" in which our needs can be met and our desires fulfilled.

> Whatever you have focused on through this process—the issue, the situation, the people, and your declaration at the end—you've released it and now you declare it done.
>
> Imagine your claim, your new intention, moving out across the planet, gathering all the resources to make it real in your experience. Then forget it, along with everything else you did today.
>
> You have released all that, and now it is no longer a part of your life or even of your story of your life. It no longer exists. In its place is your declaration, which you have put out into the world to make it so. And so it is.

Step Ten. Appreciation

Gratitude and appreciation are two of the most transforming energies we can experience. Like meditation, they improve blood flow, harmonize heart beat, improve digestion, and clarify thought. In many spiritual traditions, they are considered indications of connection with the divine. In New Thought, they are essential components of every prayer process, based on Jesus' prayer at Lazarus' tomb, in which he gave thanks for Lazarus' delivery before there was any sign it had happened. The shamanic traditions start and end each day and each ritual with expressions of deep gratitude for the things and people of this life and the support of the other energies in the universe on our paths.

> Look around at all the beauty and life that fills the world. Enjoy it. Appreciate it. You may even feel grateful for some of it—go ahead; it'll do you good. Bask in the delight of it for a while; you deserve it!
>
> If you're having difficulty seeing what to be grateful for, practice: look at a flower, an animal, a child, and think of how wonderful it is and how much richer your life is because of it. Think about the people you love and who love you, the work or pastimes that you enjoy, the beauty in your life, memories of times you were happy. Even if you can think of only one memory to appreciate or see only one thing in your life to be grateful for, you will have begun to transform your experience by focusing on that for a while.
>
> Now expand those thoughts and memories. Imagine other situations that you could appreciate and be grateful for. Imagine what it might have been like to have had different experiences. Feel the gratitude and appreciation that come with those experiences.
>
> Do this as often as possible. Remember only those things you appreciate. Talk about only those things you enjoy. Express gratitude to everyone for everything they contribute to your life.

Step Eleven. Cancel That Old Thought!

In Buddhist tradition, the mind is the source of all obstruction and dis-stress. The mind is tricky and likes to follow old grooves—even when it knows they don't really exist anymore. So we meditate; we still the mind and release the thoughts. But we can't always be in the stillness, and occasionally, as we're driving or washing dishes or taking out the garbage, the old thought pattern starts up. Sometimes it happens when we're talking with a friend. The old pattern of thought starts up and we hear words coming out of our mouth that we know we no longer believe. So we continue to train the mind in the new pattern: we cancel the old thought and replace it with a new one (which happens to be the meaning of "New Thought").

When you realize you're thinking some of those same old ungrateful or upsetting thoughts again, simply say,

"Cancel that!

It's not true!

I don't believe that!"

Then say what you know to be true. Affirm what you have declared and claimed. Whenever you start to think in the old way, after you've canceled the thought, remind yourself of your declaration. It's what's true for you now. Everything else is just a story you heard somewhere: a movie, a dream, a faded memory of someone else's life. This declaration, this claim, is all that's real, and so it's all you need to focus on for the foreseeable future.

An effective action at this stage is to go through whatever keepsakes, photos, writings, or mementos you have from the situation you've released. Notice how you feel, now, when you look at them. Toss away any that reinforce the story you've just released, and take out one or two of the others that reinforce your new, appreciative feelings. Keep them where you can see them for a while. Remind yourself of your declaration whenever you see them.

The mind will get the message after a while and stop pestering you.

Step Twelve. Stand Firm

People who have used this method are amazed at how much things change, and how quickly. As the mind-body system is transformed, experience must change as well. People who were involved in the situation we've released behave differently. Our response to similar situations is different, too.

As we've moved through these steps, we've built a strong foundation for faith in a new kind of experience, a transformed life. Now we can carry that faith forward, knowing that, at some point, we will be faced with similar situations again—but they won't have nearly the power or impact on us because we've done this work.

Faith means standing firm in the face of contrary appearances or tendencies. When we've truly done this process—acknowledging the situation, expressing until there's nothing more to say, releasing, holding the conversation, and feeling the forgiveness, then claiming a new way of being that we know is the best we can imagine for ourselves and everyone else—then we've eliminated at least 80 percent of the issue from our consciousness and life. Therefore, we can have faith that we can deal with it when it comes up again.

As life goes around on its spiral path, the situation is likely to emerge again—or something very much like it.

When you realize you're going through it again, simply repeat this process—you'll get rid of another 80+ percent, so it'll take that much less time and that much less upset before you wake up and do it again—and that much less effort to complete the process.

You'll know you're totally done with this particular pattern when you realize one day that a related event went right on by—and you didn't get hooked! Congratulations!

The method described here has been used for almost two decades by many people addressing all kinds of conditions. It can be applied to any situation that needs healing, because virtually all conditions are the result of an energy block or misalignment in the mind-body system, and our thoughts and emotions are typically what hold those blocks or misalignments in place. It works wonderfully for relationships but is just as effective for the physical symptoms that have built up through years of unhealthy emotional or physical activity, or for self-sabotaging behaviors, or just about any pattern of thinking or activity that doesn't seem to work for you. One way to think about life is, "If it doesn't feel like Paradise, it's an opportunity to release something."

References

Bateson, Gregory. *Steps to an Ecology of Mind*. New York: Ballantine, 1972.

A Course in Miracles. Wisconsin Dells, WI: A Course in Miracles International, 2005.

Miller, Ruth. *Unveiling Your Hidden Power*. Beaverton, OR: Wise-Woman Press, 2005.

Tolle, Eckhart. *The Power of Now*. Novato, CA: New World Library, 1999.

CHAPTER 13

The Healing Practice
of Humor

A merry heart does good like a medicine, but a broken spirit
dries the bones.—Proverbs 17:22

AMERICANS ENCOUNTERED A WHOLE NEW WAY of thinking about
medicine in the late 1970s when Norman Cousins, a well-
known author and former editor of the popular magazine *The Saturday Review*, published his *Anatomy of an Illness as Perceived by the
Patient*. Almost a year on the best-seller lists, the publication of that
book could well be considered the coming-of-age of holistic medicine in this country. It had such an impact that Cousins was
appointed to the faculty of the medical school at the University of
California at Los Angeles.

In August 1964, Cousins came home from a business trip with a
fever and, as he described it, "a general feeling of achiness. Within
a week it became difficult to move my neck, arms, hands, fingers,
and legs" (Cousins 1981, 28). He was diagnosed with *ankylosing
spondylitis*, a severe inflammation and disintegration of the connective tissue in and around the spine, with one chance in five hundred of recovery. Pain and paralysis quickly overwhelmed him,
and he was hospitalized.

Exploring possible origins for his illness, Cousins came to the conclusion that his adrenal glands and endocrine system had been severely overtaxed.

> I knew well that the full functioning of my endocrine system—in particular the adrenal glands—was essential for combating severe arthritis or, for that matter, any other illness.... I remembered having read ... that adrenal exhaustion could be caused by emotional tension ... The inevitable question arose in my mind: ... If negative emotions produce negative chemical changes in the body, wouldn't the positive emotions produce positive chemical changes? (ibid., 34)

He explored a number of possibilities with his doctor and came up with his own prescription: eating more nutritious foods, increasing the level of ascorbic acid (vitamin C) in his body, and eliminating all toxic medications, even to control pain. To encourage positive emotions and relieve pain, Cousins focused on feeling love, faith, and hope as much as possible, and sought out ways to laugh more.

> A good place to begin, I thought, was with amusing movies.... It worked. I made the joyous discovery that ten minutes of genuine belly laughter had an anesthetic effect and would give me at least two hours of pain-free sleep. (ibid., 39)

He began watching humorous films and laughing uproariously every few hours. However, the sounds from his "treatments" were disturbing other patients, so he moved out of the hospital and into a hotel.

> At the end of the eighth day I was able to move my thumbs without pain.... it seemed to me that the nodules on my neck and the backs of my hands were beginning to shrink. There was no doubt in my mind that I was going to make it back all the way. I could function, and the feeling was indescribably beautiful. (ibid., 43)

Over the next several months, he steadily improved. As he was writing the book, a dozen years later, "I have become pain-free, except for one shoulder and my knees, although I have been able to discard the metal braces. I can ride a horse flat out and hold a camera with a steady hand ..." (ibid., 43)

Research Results

The human race has only one really effective weapon, and that's laughter. The moment it arises, all our hardnesses yield, all our irritations and resentments slip away, and a sunny spirit takes their place.—Mark Twain

Cousins' work opened a new door in medicine. Soon after, psychiatrist Frank Lawlis found that when patients in his pain clinics were asked what factors were the most significant in their recovery, humor was often mentioned. For example: "Once I begin to laugh, my pain starts to recede and I can see life from a different perspective" (1996, 178). Lawlis quotes several studies from the late 1980s, measuring the effects of laughter.

... people who responded to the comedy did have higher concordant EEG readings compared with those who did not ... (Svebak 1986, 133) ... Results of another study suggest that a good belly laugh can prompt the brain to block manufacture of immune suppressors ... or speed up production of immune enhancers. (Long 1987) ... Another researcher concluded that laughter increases breathing activity and oxygen exchange, increases muscular activity and heart rate, and stimulates [various] system[s] ... (Lawlis 1996, 183–84)

There are two stages of response in laughter: an arousal phase, with increased physiological parameters, and a resolution phase, when the parameters return to resting rate or lower. In the arousal stage, a number of muscle groups become active: diaphragm, abdominal, intercostal, respiratory, accessory, facial, and occasionally in the arms, legs, and back. In vigorous, sustained laughter, the heart rate is stimulated, sometimes reaching rates above 120 beats per minute. The breathing pattern becomes chaotic, with respiratory rate and depth increased, while volume is decreased, so oxygen saturation of peripheral blood is not significantly changed, in spite of the increased ventilation and the increased peripheral blood flow occurring during sustained laughter. As most of us know, too well, coughing and hiccups are often triggered by laughter—due to phrenic nerve irritation or the dislodging of mucus plugs. As a result, conditions such as asthma or bronchitis may be irritated by vigorous laughter.

Clearly, laughter affects the mind-body in significant ways. The question is, how? Lawlis suggests several possibilities. Humor coming as a change shifts the mind-body in significant ways. It reduces tension in the body and suffering in the mind. It changes the person's energetic field. There are neurological and hormonal benefits. The energy field of the body increases in flow. The mind-body should liven up.

Paul McGhee, in *Health, Healing, and the Amuse System* (1996), reports that, as a result of these activities, the following benefits accrue:

- Muscle Relaxation: Belly laughs result in muscle relaxation. While you laugh, the muscles that do not participate in the belly laugh, relax. After you finish laughing those muscles involved in the laughter start to relax. So, the action takes place in two stages.

- Cardiac Exercise: A belly laugh is equivalent to "an internal jogging." Laughter can provide good cardiac conditioning especially for those who are unable to perform physical exercises.

- Blood Pressure Reduction: Women seem to benefit more than men in preventing hypertension through laughter.

• Respiration Enhancement: Frequent belly laughter empties your lungs of more air than is taken in, resulting in a cleansing effect similar to deep breathing, especially beneficial for patients who are suffering from emphysema and other respiratory ailments.

Studies through the late 1980s and early '90s suggested even more positive effects of laughter on the immune system. Drs. Lee Berk and Stanley Tan of Loma Linda University in California have shown that laughing lowers blood pressure, reduces stress hormones, increases muscle flexion, and boosts immune function by raising levels of infection-fighting T-cells, disease-fighting proteins called gamma interferon, and B-cells, which produce disease-destroying antibodies. They found that laughter also triggers the release of endorphins, the body's natural painkillers, and produces a general sense of well-being. And Kathleen Dillon at Western New England College demonstrated an increased concentration of salivary IgA, another indicator of an enhanced immune system, in subjects who viewed a humorous video (Dillon 1985, 1).

So, truly, as *The Reader's Digest* regularly reminds us, laughter is "the best medicine." Hearing a good joke, a fun comedian, or a well-timed pun, having a "giggle session" with family or friends, watching a funny play, movie, or television show—all contribute to our overall health and well-being and can provide temporary relief from suffering.

Laughter and Meditation

B UT LAUGHTER DOES EVEN MORE. According to well-known physician and author, Larry Dossey (Lawlis 1996, 191), the studies suggest that laughter and deep meditation have much in common. Both laughter and meditation produce feel-good endorphins, but the psychological freedom that comes from laughter and meditation is a deeper joy. They both help us go beyond what seems to be our personal limitations. Both meditation and laughter bring us into transpersonal resource. Both help us shift from self-centeredness into the unlimited transpersonal realm. The laughter response, by increasing blood flow, shifting our focus away from "normal reality," and offering a different perspective from which to look at the world, is a delightful addition to any healing method.

Guidelines for Inducing Laughter

EARLIER WE SUGGESTED that illness is a state of consciousness. We pointed out that, regardless of the specific symptoms, certain patterns of thought and feeling are consistent across the spectrum of illness. The implication of that statement is that any practice that shifts us from the state of consciousness called Illness will, at the least, facilitate the healing process and, at best, release the symptoms and allow us to regain health. Laughter is one of those practices.

When we laugh, we are enhancing the vitality of our own mind-body. And when we encourage others to laugh, we can do as much for others. The trick is to do so with great consideration for the audience. Offering the gift of humor, then, means paying close attention to the audience—really listening to who this person is, and seeking out ways that will surprise, please, and shift her or him. Humor can be ordinary, or a skill, or an art. A crucial factor always is the response of the audience. Amusing oneself is one thing, but making someone else laugh has a double healing value, as we shall see.

Clearly, some people have a knack for making people laugh. Others have a witty way of speaking, using clever wording, to amuse themselves and others. Most people enjoy saying things that make other people happy. It feels doubly healthy. Surprise and timing are often elements of humor, and they cause a shift that brings release. These elements are most commonly found in the standard joke structure, known as the "triple," which has three stages. First, there's the preparation, then building up anticipation, and finally, the punch line, or payoff.

The preparation is the part of the joke or story or skit that starts out perfectly normal. The status shift occurs when the situation suddenly doesn't fit our normal world. The new state is incongruous. It doesn't fit our expectations. It's outside of our norm. As the story unfolds we are held in this state of ambivalence, not quite sure what to expect, until the punch line—and release. Aaah! A classic example is:

> A nature lover is hiking on a mountain trail when he trips and sprawls and tumbles down over a ledge. As he falls, he frantically grabs some roots on the edge and finds himself dangling out in space. He quickly realizes he's in a desperate situation and calls out, with all his might, "If there's anyone out there, please help me!"
>
> Almost immediately, a voice comes out of the sky and says, "This is God speaking. Trust me. Let go and fall free. Trust me."
>
> After a couple of seconds, the guy calls out again, "Is there anyone else out there?"

If the status shift sets up a new state that is too far from our norm—or has us focusing on something we find disturbing or contrary to our morals (for example, really raunchy "dirty" jokes)—we may find ourselves laughing nervously, rather than uproariously, if we laugh at all. Which is why listening and paying attention to the audience is so important.

Another structure for humor is the "pun," or *double entendre,* in which a word is used in a surprising way, based on an alternate meaning or pronunciation. For example,

> A Native American man is suffering from anxiety. Finally, he goes to a psychotherapist. Once there, he's so beside himself that he can barely sit still.

He says, "Doc, I'm so confused. It's like one day I think I'm a wigwam, the next day I think I'm a tepee." The doctor thinks for a minute and then he says, "I see your problem. You're too tense."[20]

The pun is similar to the "reverse," in which the jokester uses a word or concept in a way that is opposite to its usual use or meaning. Stand-up comedy depends on this, as in the classic line, "Take my wife ... please!" Or it may be used in a story, as:

Two hydrogen atoms meet. One says, "I've lost my electron." The other says, "Are you sure?" The first replies, "Yes, I'm positive."

Another version of the reverse is the following:

A woman was on a long drive across the high desert when she spotted an elderly woman walking along the side of the road. Partly out of compassion and partly for the company, she stopped and offered the elder a ride.

After a moment's consideration, the elderly woman got into the car and arranged her bundles on her lap. Then they drove off together.

For the next several miles the elderly woman said nothing. She seemed preoccupied with examining everything in the car.

Finally, the woman driving noticed that her passenger was studying a paper bag that lay on the seat between them. By way of explanation, she said, "That's a bottle of wine I got for my husband."

The elderly woman nodded and said, "Good trade."

A common visual structure, especially in political cartoons and television, is called "paired elements," in which incongruous elements are put together in surprising ways. The classic Marx Brothers and

---

20. The pun is in the homophone: "two tents."

"I Love Lucy" humor was often of this type—and it was the foundation for the ongoing popularity of the television series "Friends." Jokes about the afterlife often use this device, as:

> Twin brothers, Joe and Moe, are very close family and friends, but then Joe gets very sick and is going to die. Moe says to him, "Joe, I want you to contact me from the beyond. I want to know how you're doing. I want you to reach me and tell me what it's like." Joe says, okay. He'll try.
>
> Joe dies, and some time later Moe is shocked. It's Joe's voice, like a telephone going off in his mind. He's calling from the afterlife.
>
> Moe says, "Joe, hey, tell me what it's like there!"
>
> Joe says, "Well, we get up in the morning, and we have sex. We nap a little and then we eat. Then we play for a while. Then we rest and eat some more. Then we have sex again. Then we rest."
>
> Moe says to Joe, "Wow. Heaven sounds great!"
>
> And Joe says, "Heaven? What heaven? I'm a jack rabbit in Wyoming."

In all of these structures, the essence is surprise. We laugh as a form of release, in response to an unexpected turn of events. And, although it's possible to program surprises, some of the best humor emerges spontaneously, and in the company of dearly loved friends and family, which is, of course, the best healing, by far.

The Method

CLEARLY, THE BIOLOGICAL BENEFITS of humor are impressive, and they are even more beneficial when we practice humor in order to raise the spirits of someone else. When you tell a joke or a humorous story to another person, it has a double benefit. You give your own spirit a lift in order that the joke or story has its best effect, and you get the satisfaction of lifting the spirit of another person. And, when you do it specifically to help someone who may be sick or suffering, you also get the benefits that come from being compassionate. In this sense the practice of humor to benefit another and yourself is similar to the practice of Compassionate Breathing: by benefiting another you doubly benefit yourself.

To begin practicing this method, go to a library or to a bookstore in search of collections of jokes and/or humorous stories. There are many such collections, with titles like "The World's 1,000 Best Jokes," "500 Funny Stories," "500 Great Speech Openers." In any humor collection you'll probably find at least a few jokes or stories that strike you really well. Copy those out. Memorize them and practice telling them to yourself. You'll probably find that to be fun. Then practice telling the jokes to someone you're comfortable with who is willing to be your audience. People usually at least smile and often laugh when someone tells them a joke.

Even if you've never told jokes before (which is rare among humans), you'll probably find it to be fun. People tend to love telling jokes. We get a charge out of being funny, and if you ever find that you're sick, you'll probably be practicing healing yourself with humor.

If Illness is a state of consciousness, then any method that shifts us out of that state of consciousness can help to heal. Humor is clearly one of those. We can find humor in every day, and a shared laugh can be a most healing experience. As Patch Adams and numerous hospital clowns have demonstrated, humor and healing go hand in hand.

References

Berk, Lee, and Stanley Tan. *Humor and Health Journal* (September/October 1996).

Cousins, Norman. *Anatomy of an Illness as Perceived by the Patient.* New York: Penguin, 1981.

Dillon, Kathleen. "Positive Emotional States and Enhancement of the Immune System." *International Journal of Psychiatry in Medicine* 15 (1985): 1.

Fry, William F. "Mirth and the Human Cardiovascular System." In *The Study of Humor,* Harvey Mindess and Joy Turek, eds., Los Angeles: Antioch University Press, 1979.

Lawlis, G. Frank. *Transpersonal Medicine.* Boston: Shambhala, 1996.

Long, Patricia. "Laugh and Be Well." *Psychology Today* (October 1987): 28–29.

McGhee, Paul. *Health, Healing, and the Amuse System.* New York: Kendall/Hunt, 1996.

Svebak, Sven. "The Effect of Mirthfulness upon Amount of Discordant Right-Left Occipital EEG Alpha." *Motivation and Emotion* 6, no. 2 (1986): 133–46.

CHAPTER 14

Health Care Methods for the Semi-Comatose and Comatose, and for Near-Death Care

AUDIO-GUIDANCE PROVIDES A MEANS for practicing self-care methods, regardless of the capacity of the listener to speak or act. Self-administered, the use of guided meditation processes makes it possible for anyone to achieve the healthful effects of deep meditation anywhere, without years of training or discipline. Administered to the comatose or dying, the audio-guide helps the patient maximize inner awareness to restore balance, even when outer concerns and capacities no longer seem to matter. The following methods apply the audio-guide meditation approach in a variety of settings.

Alzheimer's Care: Treatment for the Semi-Comatose

Over the past decade, Alzheimer's disease has become a significant, expensive health care problem, destroying the lives of millions of elderly individuals and placing immense stress on their families, particularly the primary caregiver. The disease progresses slowly, sometimes affecting the lives of those involved for as much as a decade. Its characteristic symptoms are:

- memory loss
- general cognitive dysfunction
- dementia
- autism
- increasing physical dysfunction

In spite of millions of dollars in research, experimentation, and treatment, Era I medicine, with its focus on the chemistry and physiology of the body and brain, has failed to either prevent or treat this sadly debilitating condition.

However, the potential for healing through direct access to inner awareness is great. By focusing on the function that underlies all mental processes, it's possible to reduce, and even reverse, many symptoms. The torment many patients feel, knowing that they can't speak or think as they used to or want to, can be released as they turn away from trying to deal with the outer world and turn inward to inner awareness, to the deep, inner knowing in the nonverbal, transpersonal domain.

The following remarkable true story is an inspiration for our approach to Alzheimer's therapy. Published in *Kitchen Table Wisdom,* by Rachel Naomi Reman (1997), the story is told by a doctor, Tim, about his father. About ten years before his death, Tim's father had become silent and then progressively more passive and helpless, requiring constant care. One day, Tim's mother had gone shopping and Tim and his brother, fifteen and seventeen years old, respectively, were watching a football game on TV, with their father seated in a chair nearby. Suddenly, there was a loud crash. Their father had fallen forward heavily onto the floor. His face was gray; they knew something was seriously wrong. Tim told his brother to call 911. Then a voice they hadn't heard for ten years said, "Don't call 911, son. I'm all right. Tell your mother that I love her." And he died (ibid., 300). Similar anecdotes about the comatose and semi-comatose abound, pointing to an inner awareness and capacity that seem impossible when brain function has so badly deteriorated. There are many such remarkable stories, and for every one that is reported, research has shown that up to a hundred similar stories go unreported.

The method we are presenting here was developed by Medi-Grace to therapeutically access inner awareness. An audio-guide is available in the MediGrace catalog as *Alzheimer's Care* (MG5). It's derived from the same basic meditation methods described earlier. It provides direct access to inner awareness through the use of an audio-guide giving instructions that have been carefully designed for shifting attention. This method has a twofold healing potential: it reduces stress and supports the inner foundation for mental and physical functioning, in both the patient and the caregiver, at the same time. Therefore, we recommend that both the patient and caregiver have regular and frequent opportunities to listen to the audio-guide—the more the better for the highest possible impact.

THE METHOD

Inner Peace
(Alzheimer's Care)

Following is a condensed version of the audio-guide transmission of the method. You can obtain the audio-guide and
experience the method through audio-guidance.

The Practice

And so we sit here, quietly,
breathing.
Let's breathe together.
Let's be quiet together.
Let's feel the energy
in the inner quiet.
Let's learn peace.

Let's breathe together.
Let's have this quiet.
Let's learn peace.

Teach me to communicate
with you in a new way.
Teach me to know
your wisdom inside.

Teach me to know
the inner way.
Send me energy from your inner mind.
Communicate
with your telepathic mind.

Let me hear you
without listening.
Let me know you
without thinking.
Let me see you
without looking.

Reach me
from deep inside you.
Reach me
with the energy of deep life.

Teach me
to be telepathic.
Teach me
to see
with new eyes.

Let's see together
as one.
Let's see
as if we're seeing all life.
Let's see the light in our bodies.
Let's see the light
in our minds.

Teach me
without words
how to really know.

Communicate
without words
what I need to know.

What is here
alive
in our presence?

What is here
beating alive
in our hearts?

Heal me
and heal with me
into grace.

Now is the time
to turn into
the source of life.

This is what
we've been living for.

Care for me
and teach me how to care.

Feel the whole world
become peaceful in us.

Could it be
that we hold
the key to peace?

Let's love life now
like we never could.

Now is the time
for all the world
to touch sacred ground.

Can it be that this is
the moment in time
we've been living for?

Without words
show me inside
the way to all life.

Let's be silent now
so we'll be able to
come to life anew.

You will speak again
as if you've learned to say
what life needs to hear.

Let us go
so far into life
we'll come into the presence
of all of life.
The deeper we go
the more we see
there's nothing to fear.

Let's be alive
in this secret place
to realize peace,
joy and peace.

Sit with me now.
Breathe with me now.
Let me stay with you.

Let's bless the world.
Let's be in peace.

Healing Through Hearing
in Unconscious States

I N ALTERED STATES SUCH AS COMA, the patient may be, or seem to
be, "stuck" in an impenetrable isolation. But since the West has
discovered inner awareness and the possibilities associated with
nonlocal mind (Dossey 1989), many of us have shifted our attention to the inner awareness of those in such states, beginning to
explore ways to reach people who once were believed to be unreach-
able. In some cases, we are able to help them shift attention suffi-
ciently to break out of states that have locked them away from the
outer world. As Arnold Mindell observes,

> We are less concerned with recovering expression or move-
> ment than with facilitating inner release and realization . . .
> refine methods to help people in altered states connect to
> their own inner awareness. (1989, 5)

Understanding this possibility, and on the basis of the research
concerning awareness-based meditation techniques, MediGrace
has developed an audio-guide, *Healing Through Hearing in Unconscious States* (MG2, Side A), combining music and language to help
people in altered states develop their capacity to function in inner
awareness. Designed to reach inner awareness and offer the possibility of inner release, or even realization and liberation, the audio-
guide may be used in routine nursing care or in-home care. This
audio-guide is most effective when played at a soft, but audible
sound level, near the patient's head.

We can be confident in the knowledge that there are ways to
guide people in profoundly altered states, such a coma, to a new
sense of life and possibility.

The Method

Healing Through Hearing
in Unconscious States

Following is a version of the audio-guide transmission of the method. You can obtain the audio-guide and experience the method through audio-guidance.

The Practice

It's always been the time of miracles every moment.
It's hot life on electric Earth.
We're blazed and tested by the light of life.
We're blazed and tested by the light of death.
Some come through like diamond, deathless.
Others turn away from their light.
Some break all the interference patterns,
and the great life dynamic realizes itself.
The life force is healed in all being.
The new world changes in the living.
Force is the world we see change.

This is music for a new kind of eyesight.
This is music for a new kind of speech.
This is music for a new kind of life.
You can hear it in the action you beat.
You can go into the goodness of your light.
There's no stopping the world from evolving.
There's no stopping the life the new world has to give.
Earth is absolutely charged with life,
and it pulses with the charge into space.

This is music for a new charge of life.
This is music for a new vital blaze.
Come to life
awaking within.
Blaze with life
reemerging inside.
Now is the time. Now is the time.

It's always been the time of the miracles of life.

It's always been the time of the miracles of death.
We're always tested by the light of life.
We're always tested by the light of death.
Some come through to great life gain.
Others turn away from their light.
Some break through all interference
and the flesh dynamic realizes life itself.
The force of it heals all being.
This is compassion of the clear light field.
Now is the time to know.
Now is the time for greater life.
This is music for new life in your body.
This is music for new life in your mind.

The action in your cells changes fields.
You come clear in the live charge of your heart.
You are more and more charged with life.
You pulse with the charge to awake.

This is music for a new charge of life.
This is music to awake the state.
Come to life
gaining charge.
Come to blaze
receiving life.

Awake at last,
awake for good,
once and for all.

Healing in Near-Death Care

THE HOSPICE CARE MOVEMENT emerged at the end of the twentieth century, during the height of Era I medicine—an era that has been characterized by the intense use of drugs, machines, and other medical techniques to intervene in and extend the final stages of bodily life. With the emerging Era III understandings of the non-local effects of practices such as the Buddhist *Tong Len* (see Chapter Ten), hospices now can offer new possibilities for people completing the life cycle.

Meditation-based near-death care prepares people for the powerful experiences they will encounter as the body begins to shut down, and offers new ways to help people previously thought to be out of reach achieve new levels of capability. Audio-guidance in near-death states can facilitate inner awakening and the realization of deathless states as the body seems to be letting go of life. The MediGrace audio-guide *Near Death Care / After Death Care* (MG2, Side B) may be self-administered or administered by a caregiver. Potential applications for this method include:

- people doing healing work while asleep (self-administered)
- people who are bedridden and largely unconscious or comatose due to late stages of a disease (administered)
- people whose brains have been traumatized (administered)
- people preparing for death or rebirth (administered and self-administered)

This audio-guide method may be used for inner development at any time in life, or in hospice care. It may be applied in routine nursing care, or in-home care, or in a hospice. It is applied to the incapacitated person at soft but audible sound levels near the person's head. The combination of voice and sacred sound is intended to awaken inner awareness and offer the possibility of inner release or even realization and liberation.

Though words in the audio-guide call those who will hear them to "come to life," to "regain life," it's to be understood from the way it's being said that the text is not necessarily calling for people to awaken from comatose states, or to reverse states of dying, and arise. If that happens, good; if not, a level of healing and inner release may still have occurred. The "life" that the recorded voice is calling one into is life beyond physical life and death, the inherent awakened state, what Mindell calls "the immortal you." "Life after death appears as a timeless eternal reality trying to manifest itself in the present" (1989, 4). Death can be a healing into greater life, as many have known.

Liberation Through Hearing During and After Death

AFTER DEATH WE CAN HEAR in two ways. We not only hear very clearly, because the mental body has all the faculties of the physical body, but we telepathically know the meaning of the sacred texts that may be read to us. We are able to practice the teachings as we hear them.

The MediGrace audio-guide *Liberation Through Hearing After Death* (MG2, Side B) is a concise presentation of the renowned text: *The Tibetan Book of the Dead* ("The Great Liberation Through Hearing in the Bardo"). The words invoke awareness directly, instructing us to realize our light, now and in the after-death states. They are offered before and after death, understanding that, even after death, we have chance after chance to come alive: awakening to awareness at any time—even in altered states of being—is the transformative process.

The audio-guide gives the famous sacred instructions for dying and for progress in the after-death states. The program has been edited for general use in homes and in hospices. It is administered at a low, but audible volume, either with headphones or speakers placed very near the head. The program begins with an introduction to the Tibetan text.[21] Then the music begins, an ancient music for many instruments, great horns and drums, issuing harmonies of this and all worlds. It makes a timeless field for the melodic chanting of the revered instructions, teachings known to liberate when they are heard.

This is a melodic energy medicine applied when conventional, Era I medicine can only obscure, distress, or disturb natural processes that could lead to transformation or transcendence. This method gives us something valuable to offer to those who are dying and those who have just passed on.

---

21. The Tibetan text is a famous revelation of Padmasambhava, who brought *Vajrayana* Buddhism to Tibet in the eighth century. It's a major subject of Sogyal Rinpoche's *The Tibetan Book of Living and Dying*.

The Method

Liberation Through Hearing During and After Death

Following is a version of the audio-guide transmission of the method. You can obtain the audio-guide and experience the method through audio-guidance.

Introduction

And so you will come to the death of your physical body,
your time to enter a new state of being.
Let's make an offering of music,
awakened music,
and let's hear the sacred instructions,
called *Liberation Through Hearing After Death.*

The Practice

During the time of life in this human body
few people succeed in waking up.
In physical death and in states after that
we have chance after chance to come alive.
This is what ancient wisdom is saying.
Before and after death listen to the sacred instructions.

We have the chance to awaken again and again after death.

After physical death we're much more clairvoyant, more in touch
    with light.
After death we have great understanding and knowing.
After we die we can
read the mind of a living person.
We can hear telepathically,
understanding the meaning of a text read to us,
even if we've never heard the language before.
The ancient wisdom says that in states after death
the mental body has the faculties of the sense body.
We're told that we can see and hear intently after death.
We can be invoked to hear and realize the wisdom teachings.
But just as intensely our mind projects and interferes.

The great challenge after death is to recognize mind
to be much more aware.
So prepare to be awake as your body dies,
awake in death.
Recognize mind.
Be ready to receive omniscient teachings.
Be ready to know all your fears and be free.
So now, at whatever moment of your life
you can use teaching on how to recognize mind,
and how to act for the benefit of all life.
Especially when we're close to the time of death,
in order to prepare for the intensity of being disembodied,
or if we are now in an after-death state,
hear the music and the voice of the wisdom teachings.

Hear and become liberated for the benefit of all life.

The healing that occurs with these methods is not always visible to the eye but is always felt. As we observe those who are no longer able to communicate with us verbally moving through these practices, we can often see them relax into a new state of being, but even if we don't *see* the changes, we can *feel* them. Those we love and care for are no longer separate from us; they are part of the energy body we are. As we still our minds and sense, with our energy body, the energy body of the one whose manifest body is so still, we can feel the shift that body goes through as the truth of this ancient wisdom is perceived and accepted.

References

Jung, Carl G. *Memories, Dreams, Reflections: Life After Death*. New York: Random House, 1961.

Dossey, Larry. *Recovering the Soul*. New York: Bantam, 1989.

Mindell, Arnold. *Coma: Key to Awakening*. Boston: Shambhala, 1989.

Reman, Rachel. *Kitchen Table Wisdom*. New York: Riverhead/Penguin-Putnam, 1997.

PART FOUR

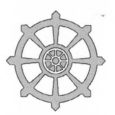

New Possibilities

CHAPTER 15

Transforming Our Paradigm of Illness

HISTORICALLY, ERA I MEDICINE has focused on applying a particular protocol to a particular individual with particular symptoms. The assumption was that, at best, that individual would be free of those symptoms and, at worst, that individual would continue to suffer or the symptoms would cause him or her to die, at which point the medical practitioner would simply try to make a patient pain-free as he or she moved through the dying process.

Yet more and more evidence tells us that this need no longer be the case.

One of the more profound consequences of using the methods outlined in Part Three of this book is that we begin to realize that our distress and pain are not burdens to bear, but opportunities to transform. As we use the breathing and the compassion and the healing processes contained in these methods, we begin to see that we are not the illness, nor the body in distress. We begin to understand that we are not the victim of some dreadful organism or circumstance or system. And, as we begin to experience freedom from all these limited perceptions, we begin to move through and beyond the symptoms that required us to stop and use the methods in the first place.

In Chapter Four, we suggested that Illness is a state of consciousness. We outlined some of the characteristics of that state, including the fact that people tend to become passive, rather than active, moving in and out of sleeping/dreaming more frequently than in "normal" waking consciousness or sleep. Interestingly, it is in these characteristics that the opportunity for transformation of consciousness is found.

As we find ourselves less active, we are more willing to relax. As we find ourselves more "dreamy" and less "focused," we are more willing to simply observe our breathing and the thoughts that move through our awareness. As we feel more discomfort in our bodies, we are more willing to find ways to release the sensation. As we drift into the inner dimensions of semi-coma, we process and release the past with fewer distractions from the present.

Western scientific medicine has seen these characteristics of illness as symptoms to be treated or, at best, stages in the healing process. Eastern traditions have, for the most part, done likewise. Across time and cultures, only the shamanic traditions, based on the understanding that all of life is a balancing of interacting forms of consciousness, have treated Illness as a state of consciousness to be transformed by the practitioner. In our culture, only "faith healers" and Christian Science or New Thought practitioners have done so. The fact that this approach works more often than not has not prevented Western science from calling such practitioners "witch doctors" and "charlatans," simply because the observed results haven't fit the scientific paradigm.

Today, however, with the new understandings of how matter and energy are formed and transformed, and with the undeniable results of thousands of experiments showing the nonlocal nature of mind, it is no longer wise to discount the effectiveness of such approaches to Illness. So Western researchers are in the middle of a scientific revolution—a shift from a paradigm of analysis and deductive reasoning toward a paradigm of holism and intuitive understanding.

Fortunately, a few experts in the "new" paradigm remain. A few "medicine men and women" and "holy men and women" and *swamis* and *yogis* and lamas and shamans have managed to continue their practice and teaching in ways that Westerners can learn and benefit from.

We have relied on these teachings for this book. Our model of the human mind-body as outlined in Chapter Five and the methods suggested for use in Part Three are derived and integrated from both the new sciences and the ancient wisdom.

And, as we have done so, we've seen our own understanding transformed. For we, like so many others in our culture, had tended to see Illness as something to avoid, something to heal and move on from. But as we worked with and practiced and thought about our experience with these ideas and the methods, we came to understand that, through the experience of Illness, each of us (and the people around us) had gone through a transformative process.

One way to look at this process is presented in C. S. Holling's ecosystems model. Holling, a biologist trying to understand the dynamics of insect infestations in forests, has described a process that applies to all living systems in distress.

According to Holling, everything starts as a seed—an idea, a dream, an egg. The seed grows and develops and becomes a seedling, a vision, or a company or an activity. This grows and includes more and more others—cells, plants, animals, or people—and begins to take on structure. The structure gets stronger and stronger: the tree no longer sways with the wind, the company no longer reacts to the market, the body no longer bounces back as quickly. Then some shift in the environment occurs. It may be major, a storm or fire or job loss, or it may be seemingly minor, like a change in the cost of a raw material or the minimum wage. But the structure is so inflexible that the change is too much. There's no easy way to respond and so it begins to fall apart. Things get chaotic. Trees fall down. Companies go under or cut way back. Bodies have high fevers or weird growths.

Then, amazingly, in the midst of the chaos, something happens. New seeds emerge (the seeds of redwood trees and some grasses

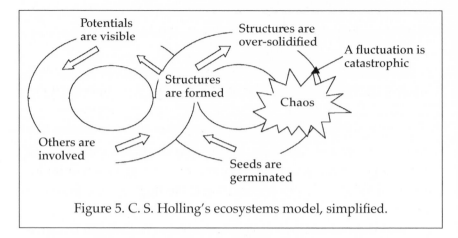

Figure 5. C. S. Holling's ecosystems model, simplified.

need fire to sprout!). New ideas can be implemented that couldn't have existed before. New relationships are formed.

So the cycle begins again. Nothing is quite the same, but the same process happens anyway—until the next "catastrophe" and ensuing "chaos" allow new seeds to form.

Illness goes through the same process. In fact, virtually every state of consciousness can be seen as going through the same process. More interestingly, however, Illness is usually seen as the "catastrophe" and the "chaos" in the process of our lives—disrupting normality with its demands and distress and too often leaving a path of destruction in its wake.

Yet if we know that this process is how life works and we think of Illness as the result of a "catastrophe" that has led to this "chaos" out of which new seeds will emerge for our lives, then a whole new set of possibilities opens up for us. Now, instead of wasting our energy being upset at the symptoms, we can be grateful for the opportunity to rest. Now, instead of being upset at the disruption of our routine, we can appreciate the new perspective that being still for a while can give us. Now, instead of trying to minimize the symptoms, we can carefully and patiently observe them to see what the mind-body is telling us through them—what kinds of needs have not been met; what kinds of actions might be taken. Now, instead of wailing about our own distress, we can use the opportunity to consider the distress of others and begin to be compassionate (from the root meaning "feeling with").

If we go beyond the immediate experience and consider how it has emerged through our history, we can see the opportunity to heal the past—and heal the present and future in the process.

If we go into the immediate present and, using methods like those presented in this book, allow ourselves to experience the depths that are possible in meditation, we can use the opportunity provided in Illness to experience pure awareness or *rigpa*, that state beyond time and space in which suffering no longer exists.

So Illness can be a transformative process, and we can be transformed through it.

CHAPTER 16

Healing the Person, Healing the Planet

O UR CULTURE HAS ENCOURAGED PEOPLE to live and work in a paradigm of isolation, believing that we are disconnected from the people and environment around us. And our approach to medicine reflected that.

Yet, the evidence is clear. As the model presented in these pages suggests, we are by no means isolated, and everything we do is affected by and affects everyone around us.

The Transpersonal Mind-Body

H OW IT IS THAT what one person thinks or feels can affect another's sense of well-being has been a focus of interest for humanity throughout the history of Western culture. Because we, unlike most other cultures, believe that each human being is isolated and separate from everyone else by our skin, the mechanism for transpersonal processes has historically eluded our scientific thinkers. In cultures that see each human being as part of a universal "web of life" or "spirit," this is not a problem: what is experienced anywhere within the web is communicated everywhere—one simply has to learn how to read the signs.

Lacking such a perspective, and required by the traditions of science to use only measurable data as indicators, Western researchers have attempted for generations to develop theories that explain what they have observed—and, often, experienced: the direct apprehension of another person's thought or feeling. Typically, as in the Western esoteric tradition, they have found it impossible to do so within the scientific-materialist paradigm. As Alan Watts stated in one of his last seminars, "We spend the first year of our life learning that the self ends with our skin and the rest of our life trying to unlearn it."

As we have seen, however, the field of transpersonal studies has offered a number of scientifically validated descriptions of the transpersonal experience. Transpersonal researchers have demonstrated beyond question that people and events can affect our thoughts, emotions, and even our illnesses without physical interaction—even at a distance. As Michael Murphy so thoroughly documented in *The Future of the Body*, hundreds of experiments and research results support the realization that there are dimensions of the human experience that transcend the limitations of the physical, material body.

Rupert Sheldrake's recent work, described in *The Sense of Being Stared At* (2006), is an attempt to apply the rules of controlled experiments to the anecdotal observations of thousands of people who have responded to his requests. He has demonstrated statistically that people are aware when someone focuses attention and perception toward them, and that they can frequently tell when someone is about to telephone or email them.

Itzhak Bentov, in his *Stalking the Wild Pendulum*, offers an explanation. Based on the model of the mind-body system as a set of overlapping wave-forms, he suggests

> As our "observers," or information waves, are periodically expanding into the inner torus of the universe, so are the "observers," or information waves, of everybody else. For a tiny fraction of a second we form an information hologram with them, and this is repeated many times a second.... our

psyches, which contain all our knowledge, expand periodically into that space for a very short period of time at prac-
tically infinite velocities. There the human psyches form an
interference pattern with the psyches of all other consciousnesses in the universe. This interference pattern, or hologram
of knowledge-information, we can call the "universal mind."
... We can't separate global mind from universal mind ...
(1977, 147–48)

This has profound implications for understanding the nature of
interpersonal interaction. The energy field of, for example, a teacher
or healer with whom we resonate may affect our own fields with
healing and integrative energy that interacts with ours to create a
new level of functioning—which is the traditional explanation for
darshan or *satsang* in the Hindu tradition of teaching and learning.
In another case, the energy field of a family member, co-worker, or
supervisor that is not in resonance with our own can negatively
affect our mood and, sometimes, our level of functioning.

It also has implications for understanding our own experience of
self. If "who I am" is affected by the thoughts and feelings of those
around me—and those distant from me whose energy fields in
some way resonate with my own—then what is "who I am"? Can
I consider myself a separate individual?

Transpersonal therapists say "No." They see what perennial wisdom has been seeing, that our personal life is limited, and constantly changing, but our transpersonal life is unlimited and healed
in the great unified field. In this aspect, the transpersonal model is
very like the Buddhist model, with its *Dharmakaya* and *Sambhogakaya*
bodies as aspects of the human mind-body experience. It's also very
much in alignment with the "fields within fields" model of human
energetic systems that we described earlier. Clearly, an integration
of these models is possible.

An Interconnected Whole

Although the tools and ideas of *The Whole Earth Catalog* (1969–1985) planted the seeds of a sustainable global culture in the popular mind, Theodore Roszak's *Person/Planet* (1979) was perhaps the first description of the practical implications of living in a media-based "global village." Fritjof Capra followed soon after with his *The Web of Life* (1996), which provided a systems-based framework for understanding the interconnected organism that is the biosphere. Rupert Sheldrake has continued to develop his work with Morphic Resonance since the original publication of *A New Science of Life* (1981), as well, suggesting that some form of information field surrounds the planet, affecting the tendencies of events at the levels of the organism and cells.

Through these and many other syntheses of ideas and theories, we can observe a rich pattern of field-based understandings emerging, helping us see that we cannot be isolated.

Quantum Relationship

Another approach to understanding the nature of our interconnectedness has emerged from the field of quantum physics. Though the work and ideas of Fred Alan Wolfe *(Space-Time and Beyond; Quantum Reality)*, Nick Herbert *(Quantum Reality)*, and Brian Greene *(The Elegant Universe)* are perhaps best known, a remarkable series by Oxford physicist-philosopher Danah Zohar provides another, useful perspective. Zohar, whose husband is a psychotherapist, was writing books explaining quantum processes when she became pregnant. As she went through the process of nurturing the life within her, she became aware that she was no longer able to identify herself as an isolated individual. She had to acknowledge that her identity was no longer that of an isolated entity but was a function of her relationships. She proceeded to write *Quantum Self* (1990), which was soon followed by *Quantum Society* (1995) and later, with her husband, *SQ: Connecting with Our Spiritual Intelligence* (2001).

Zohar's thesis is that the fundamental units that make up all matter and energy in the universe are neither matter nor energy but, in fact, tendencies for relating. These minute "wavicles," far smaller than electrons or even photons, emerge and then disappear into and out of nowhere. One of these, the *boson* (named after Satyendra Nath Bose, the physicist from India who partnered with Einstein to describe the Bose-Einstein condensate,[22] which is the basis for superconductivity), Zohar says is the tendency to come together. The second, the *fermion* (named after the Italian American who led the Manhattan Project that first split the atom, Enrico Fermi), is the tendency to move apart. Everything, she says, is made up of these two manifestations of the quantum vacuum, interacting in a dynamic balancing act through the formation of energy and matter. Individually and together, she suggests, they demonstrate a rudimentary form of intelligence that is present everywhere, always, throughout the universe and increases with the complexity of the system they compose. She calls this intelligence, or consciousness, "panpsychism" and offers a model of life that is made up of increasingly complex, interrelated fields of energy-based consciousness, whose patterns center on apparently individual organisms that exist, in fact, only in terms of their interrelatedness with other patterns of energy / consciousness.

Itzhak Bentov, coming from another perspective, agrees:

> Matter contains / is consciousness. Our planet is therefore a larger consciousness, and so is the sun. A rudimentary consciousness contained in matter and living cells maintains the

---

22. A Bose-Einstein condensate is the form of matter that is so tightly interconnected that action at any point immediately affects the whole. It has traditionally been believed that such things could exist only at super-cold temperatures but the characteristics have recently been observed in the human body and other "normal" circumstances.

life in the body. A higher consciousness, the human psyche, inhabits that body most of the time but is also independent of it. (1977, 147–48)

A somewhat different approach is offered by theoretical physicist Amit Goswami, in his *The Self-Aware Universe* (1993) and in the film *What the BLEEP Do We Know!?* Goswami suggests that it is not the "wavicles" or particles that demonstrate intelligence, but the very field out of which they emerge and of which they are, necessarily, a part. Drawing on Hindu *Vedic* literature for descriptive language, Goswami uses the image of "Indra's Net" to describe the field of consciousness that, he suggests, is the underlying framework for all existence and is exhibited throughout space and time.

In all these quantum-mechanical approaches, two fundamental understandings are consistent, based on the experimental evidence. First, the fundamental units of the universe exhibit the fundamental quality of intelligence: they *choose* which form they shall take, based on the structure of the system in which they are generated, including the thought processes of those observing the process. Second, all of these fundamental units of matter and energy exhibit a characteristic called nonlocality. That is, whenever any one of these "wavicles" is connected with another one, it will always, instantaneously, respond as if it were still connected—no matter how far apart they are in space and time. And, as we stated earlier in this text, the wave-form of energy is not limited to one point but extends throughout all space and time, all at once, overlapping with all other wave-forms in complex resonating patterns.

These two characteristics, intelligence and nonlocality, pervade all of matter and energy in all its forms, and their ubiquitous presence means that, literally, no action can occur without a parallel response, elsewhere in the universe. Quantum mechanics demonstrates, then, that intelligence is truly omnipresent and that every thought or action is instantaneously felt, everywhere.

When we realize that no one is an isolated individual, that who we are is a function of the relationships in which we participate, that we are all connected through a remarkably complex system of interacting energy fields, and that it's impossible to "do just one thing," or act in isolation, we realize that to heal any one person of any one condition, including ourselves, is to increase the likelihood of healing for all others who have that condition, as well. And the reverse. The patterns of resonance work instantly, everywhere.

Global Consciousness

One of the most amazing graphs ever produced was published on the Internet by the Global Consciousness Project at Princeton University (http://noosphere.princeton.edu) in late September 2001. Generated by a computer, this graph is one of a continuing series of integrations of reports from thirty computers around the world, connected through the World Wide Web. These computers do two things: they generate random lists of numbers and they report back to the central computer the numbers that are generated.

Normally, the report looks like a small, squiggly line, moving back and forth across zero. There's very little variation in the randomness of the numbers being generated. What made this particular graph so amazing, however, was that at 9 a.m. (Princeton time) on a particular date—September 11, 2001—the line spiked off the page. As the Twin Towers collapsed in Manhattan, the numbers generated by computers all over the world were far from random.

Even more amazing, the line had actually begun to spike several days before that date and continued to spike at lower levels for the next couple of days, dipping well below zero during the worldwide "three minutes of silence" at noon on Friday, the 14th.

What happened here?

Computer programs called random number generators produce series of numbers that usually are totally random: no pattern, no formula, can describe their relationships. It has been demonstrated thousands of times that someone sitting in front of a computer can, by changing his or her thoughts and feelings, create a pattern in

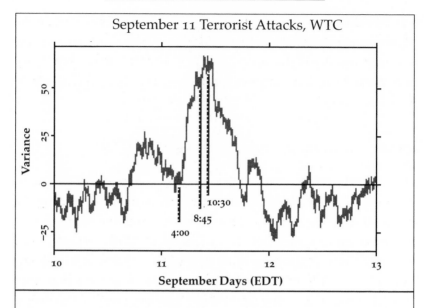

Figure 6. Graph produced by the Global Consciousness Project computers at Princeton University in September 2001. It shows the variation from randomness that occurred September 10–13, peaking when the towers were hit, then peaking again when the West Coast got the news.

the usually unrelated numbers produced on the screen by such a program. They can increase certain numbers, they can create "pictures" in the pattern that appears on the screen, they can change the output on a sheet of paper. The Consciousness Project was developed to test the hypothesis that, if one person could, then would a community or the whole of humanity be able to do so?

On 9/11, the answer came back an unequivocal "Yes." The result was that Princeton got a lot more funding for a lot more computers, and those of us who seek to understand the nature of nonlocal consciousness got a wonderful piece of data to work with.

What does the data tell us?

First, it lets us know that when people have strong thoughts or feelings, they affect the physical world in significant ways. Second, it tells us that, even before we are aware of an event, our emotions and thoughts are affected by it—in this case, even before it occurred, which is more evidence of the nonlocality of consciousness in space and *time*. Finally, it makes it clear, if it wasn't before, that, truly, nothing happens in isolation—all that we think, say, and do affects the whole world.

Prayer, Meditation, and the Maharishi Effect

Most of us have been taught that prayer is a process of asking an all-powerful divinity to give us something or make something different for us. Some of us have been taught a variation on this, based on a quote from Jesus in the New Testament: "Pray, believing you have received." A few of us have learned that prayer is an ongoing conversation with divinity, in which we express appreciation, gratitude, and praise, and through which we receive insights and deeper understandings and a peace of mind that quickly shows up in our surroundings.

Mystics from all spiritual traditions have emphasized this latter form of prayer, recognizing that through the ongoing communication with divinity, one's sense of isolation begins to dissolve and one begins to identify with the union developed through the interaction. Their resulting ecstatic experiences and visible joy have encouraged others to do the same. From Catholic saints to Hindu *gurus*, from dancing "witches" to "whirling dervishes," the mystical experience of direct communion with divinity becomes a visible radiance in the person experiencing it—inviting others to do likewise.

Prayer, however, is not the words spoken, nor even the process of interaction with the divinity.[23] Prayer is best understood as the

---

23. In the New Thought tradition, it is said that, when Jesus taught his disciples to pray, it was not the words (which is all we have to work from in the Bible), but the *manner* in which he used the words that we read—the "Our Father . . ." prayer being but a short version of the prayer that every religious Jew repeats at least once every day.

state of consciousness that results from these activities. As meta-physicians of all ages and cultures have taught, it is that state of consciousness that achieves the results—not the grace or whim of a divine being.[24]

In that state of consciousness, according to the model we've laid out in these pages, the energy fields that we are can function fully and harmoniously with, and are fully and harmoniously interacting with, all other energy fields in a resonating pattern that is manifesting our current state of consciousness. This means that, whatever we are holding in our consciousness while in this state (the state of Grace or, in Hindi *satchitananda*, "love-bliss consciousness"), whatever we *intend* is part of the totality of this harmoniously resonating pattern. This is particularly so when we understand and intend that this state is not just for us, but for all.

Two of the methods offered in these pages are explicitly designed to generate this state: "Reversal of Suffering" and 12 *Steps to Freedom*. Both of them require the practitioner to let go of whatever situation or suffering has been the focus of their attention and replace it with positive regard toward another and themselves. As they release the old way of being (the original meaning of the word "sacrifice"—from the Latin, "sacred action") and, with loving compassion, step into a new relationship with self and others, they restore harmonious function within the energy body, create new resonant harmonies with other energy fields, and, in the process, open the flow between the mind-body and the other-dimensional bodies that the Buddhists call the *trikaya*.

Other traditions have their own methods for achieving the same result. The Shaman's Journey, the Dreamtime, Spell-Casting, and the Vision Quest are a few of them, along with many of the methods of *kriya yoga*, Transcendental Meditation, and *Vajrayana* Buddhism.

Transcendental Meditation has been used and demonstrated

---

24. For a more detailed discussion of the prayer process, see Ruth Miller's *A Book of Uncommon Prayer* (2006).

statistically to be effective for reducing violence in cities and regions where a significant number (at least 1 percent) of the population is using the technique consistently (www.tm.org, 2005; *What the Bleep Do We Know!?*). This phenomenon has been labeled "the Maharishi Effect," after Maharishi Mahesh Yogi, the teacher who introduced this method to the U.S.

Whatever words are said, whatever rituals performed, the goal is to achieve that state of consciousness in which all is harmony, within Who We Are and throughout All That Is. So it is that the world is transformed.

References

Bentov, Itzhak. *Stalking the Wild Pendulum.* Rochester, VT: Destiny Books, 1977.

Brand, Stewart, et al. *The Whole Earth Catalog.* Sausalito, CA: Point Foundation, 1969–1985.

Capra, Fritjof. *The Web of Life.* New York: Anchor, 1996.

Goswami, Amit. *The Self-Aware Universe.* New York: Penguin, 1993.

Greene, Brian. *The Elegant Universe.* New York: Vintage, 1999.

Herbert, Nick. *Quantum Reality.* New York: Anchor, 1985.

Murphy, Michael. *The Future of the Body: Explorations into the Further Evolution of Human Nature.* Los Angeles: Tarcher, 1992.

Roszak, Theodore. *Person/Planet.* New York: Doubleday, 1979.

Sheldrake, Rupert. *A New Science of Life.* London: Blond & Briggs, 1981.

———. *The Sense of Being Stared At.* Los Angeles: Tarcher, 2006.

Toben, Bob, and Fred Alan Wolfe. *Space-Time and Beyond.* New York: Bantam, 1983.

Zohar, Danah. *The Quantum Self.* New York: William Morrow, 1990.

———. *Quantum Society.* London: Quill, 1995.

———, and Ian Marshall. *SQ: Connecting with Our Spiritual Intelligence.* London: Bloomsbury, 2001.

CHAPTER 17

The Genius
of Self-Care

THE GENIUS OF SELF-CARE is that the patient applies it from within, accessing inner resources that may have been previously unused. Even if the patient has intentionally used inner resources for healing to some degree in the past, he or she may not have begun to access them deeply. It's a rare person who has accessed their inner resources enough to know that they may be unlimited.

The genius of self-care is that most people can access inner resources to heal or mitigate most health conditions, and can change their lives for the better in the process. How much any individual may be able to heal a specific health problem depends on three factors: the availability of proven self-care methods; education in the use of the methods; and the quality of effort the person gives to the use of the method.

Self-care methods do exist in the public domain today. Through the unfolding of remarkable historical processes, a significant number of people on our planet, enough to make an important difference in human evolution, have access to methods that can restore healthy body function and transform consciousness. The question is: will forces of history compel the corporate medical stronghold to allow self-care into the center of the medical paradigm in the near future? We need that change soon, for the sake of human health, for the sake of the evolutionary quality of the species.

The fact that educators and the general public are asking for changes in the field of medicine based on human needs and rights is evidence of a positive historical force.

Self-care is the heart of Caroline Myss' revolutionary proposal to transfer power from the doctor to the patient (1996). It is also the essence of Herbert Benson's vision for a culture of "remembered wellness" (1996). Everyone has an inherent right to use self-care methods for general medicine, and for the transforming experiences of birth and death. Every woman has the right to be educated in advanced natural childbirth methods, self-care methods that bring out her innate ability for higher levels of prenatal and postnatal care. Everyone in the final stages of life-in-the-body has the right to be educated in near-death care methods that facilitate the transformation of consciousness as body functions cease.

It's time to call for greater education in the potential of self-care methods. Everyone has the right to be educated and trained in healing meditation methods—to experience the genius of self-care. Every man, woman, and child has the right to be educated and trained in Progressive Relaxation and deep, visualization-enhanced, optimal breathing—the essentials for well-being in all anxiety-ridden situations. It's time to propose new health care education in which people are encouraged to use self-care as a primary option. Education is the key.

Advancing Medical Options and Medical Science

I N Chapter Ten of *Timeless Healing: Optimal Medicine, Optimal Health*, Benson reintroduces

> belief-fostered healing into Western medicine. . . . the enormous cost savings that I believe can be achieved by appreciating these mind-body influences, and which have already been realized in test programs around the nation . . . (1996, 222)

At the same time, he proposes

... how medicine can make practical changes using wellness remembered across the board and reserving medications and procedures for those instances when they're needed and can be effective ... that the medicine of the future be like a three-legged stool, balanced and supported by these three components: self-care, medications, and procedures. (ibid.)

The emergence of such a development in the medical paradigm will depend on several factors:

- an increasing respect for and insistence on noninvasive methods of mind-body science, such as meditation, based on substantial research

- a willingness to inform the public about the healing potential of such methods

- the development of far-reaching education programs in self-care methods, such as meditation, throughout all levels of public and private education

- the establishment of authoritative training programs in self-care methods within the medical training institutions, including nursing schools, hospital administration programs, and the various training programs for doctors

As a species we have a great need for health care alternatives that truly empower and enhance the well-being of the individual. And, at this point in history, we have the methods. The human treasure chest of great, noninvasive meditation methods is full and accessible, so let us work together to advance the use of this benign science in all areas of health care, for the sake of all humanity.

Recently, more than 80 percent of doctors surveyed said that meditation and other mind-body methods should be studied and taught, to help establish the mind-body medical option. Yet, even now, after so much proven benefit, little progress has been made.

The evolution of the species continues to be adversely affected by the widespread use of drugs, anesthesia, and surgery. The institutionalization of birth and death worldwide has become a significant sector of the world economy—that part of the system that has been called the "health care industry." As a result, the quality of life in birth and death processes is generally reduced or obstructed.

The industrial nature of health care is perhaps most evident in the production and distribution of pharmaceuticals. Corporations with powerful lobbyists in Washington have shown a marked tendency to repress the establishment of medical alternatives to drugs, and have made an equally aggressive effort to encourage the use of pharmaceutical agents—through federal agency support and increased access to worldwide resources, media, and advertising. Recent scandals in the Food and Drug Administration simply highlight imbalances in a system that no longer works to protect consumers, but rather promotes corporate interests.

Another aspect of the "health care industry" that tends to repress nonconventional methods is the insurers. Again, large corporations with significant lobbying power work in Washington and in state legislatures to ensure that their preferred methods and procedures are supported so they may maximize stockholder returns. So, although cost reductions through mind-body medicine have been demonstrated repeatedly, the powers-that-be continue to limit access to proven methods of self-care.

Still, in spite of these deterrents, more and more people continue to learn about and choose Era II and Era III alternatives, and the body of research continues to grow—to the point where the potential of such techniques has captured the attention of the media and the medical training institutions. These noninvasive alternatives have also captured the interest of the new generation, which feels cheated and deprived of their right to a clean and healthy environment and body.

The research is conclusive: meditation practices are healing.

When we meditate, we help heal and empower ourselves. We tap the genius of self-care.

Everyone is alive by virtue of a dynamic internal life-support system, a system of vital forces and balances, and an ingenious immune system capable of producing more than 50,000 chemicals in response to internal needs, in precisely the right doses and combinations to maintain homeostasis and health. The passivity cultivated by a disempowering medical system of treatments by authority figures whose prescriptions are too often determined by corporate greed is unhealthy and deprives people of their inalienable right to choose for themselves. Noninvasive methods that work to restore balance have been proved to be far more effective in the long run than conventional medicine's interventions that simply minimize symptoms; Era II and Era III methods restore and increase health.

What the world needs is more and better health care and medical options, like teaching women about the noninvasive options in advanced natural childbirth; like offering an approach to Alzheimer's care and care for the comatose that reaches the inner awareness; like giving dying people and their loved ones a hopeful, healing process as they transition out of their bodies. The meditation methods outlined in this book are designed to do just that.

Let's finish this book with a clear statement of intent:

Realizing that intention is a powerful resource at our disposal, let's intend to benefit all humanity—past, present, and future.

Let's intend that consciousness-transforming healing methods be offered to all people, now.

May we all experience these healing benefits.

May we establish a timeless field of health everywhere on Earth.

Let self-care become planetary care.

References

Benson, Herbert. *Timeless Healing.* New York: Fireside/Simon & Schuster, 1996.

Myss, Caroline. *The Anatomy of the Spirit.* New York: Harmony Books, 1996.

Appendix:
The Light Nature of the Energy Body
According to *Vajrayana* Buddhism

Robert Bruce Newman

WE HAVE ATTEMPTED TO OFFER an integrated model of the human body that takes into account some of the profound and comprehensive knowledge of the energy body from the fields of Chinese medicine and *yoga*, in *Ayurvedic* medicine and Hindu *yoga*, as well as Tibetan medicine and *Vajrayana* Buddhist meditation science. But very little of the knowledge of the energy body in those traditions has been published. In our attempt to present a more complete model of the human body to medical science, in this book we have mentioned four kinds of *chi* functioning in the body according to Chinese medicine, and five kinds of *prana* functioning in the body according to the Hindu science of breathing. That is helpful in terms of inspiring a greater respect for the body and its subtle systems and for encouraging people to learn more about the real nature of its functions and potential.

Now, after many years of study of *Vajrayana* Buddhist meditation science it's possible to present previously unpublished information on the nature of the energy body, information confirmed through centuries of work by Tibetan meditation masters and doctors. A vision of a greatly complex body of energy channels (Tibetan: *tsa*) in which ten kinds of *prana* (Tibetan: *lung*) function, governed by light-bearing sexual essence (Tibetan: *thigle*), is summarized below, in the hope that medical science will progressively see more and more dimensions of life in the human body, and see the body as an inconceivably great form of potential.

Lung

As with *chi* and *prana*, *lung* is often translated as "air" or "wind." *Lung* originates in the primal field of the *Dharmakaya* as unconditioned life force energy. That *lung* tends to differentiate into two primal luminosities, red and white, that separate out of the clear light of the *Dharmakaya*. In a powerful conjunction of forces at the moment of human conception, awareness, integral to the red and white luminosities, enters the union of the egg and sperm (Newman, *Calm Birth*, 2005). Ten kinds of *lung* form in the first moment of body formation. Immediately three forces act together. Light-bearing cellular units of the "mother seed essence" and the "father seed essence" retain their identities as the essence of the egg and sperm and separate out in magnetic polar connection, forming the basis of the central energy channel (CEC). The white father seed essence is the brilliant point source (seed syllable) of the crown *chakra*. The red mother seed essence is the brilliant seed syllable of the navel *chakra*. These are the basis of the *thigle* of the new body. Simultaneously a total of twelve major energy channels are formed, in the moment when the ten *lungs* form and then flow in the channels. From this powerful first moment *tsa, lung,* and *thigle* are inseparable, and the *lung* and *thigle* hold the light basis of the human potential.

There are five principal *lung* movements and five subtle vital energies that derive from them. The five major *lungs* (energy winds in the body) are:

- *lung* holding the life force
- *lung* all-pervading throughout the body
- *lung* preventing deterioration (holding heat)
- upward-moving *lung* (includes digestion)
- downward-moving *lung* (includes elimination)

All five major *lungs* are held in separate ways in the CEC. When they are not held separately in a healthy way, when they "push into one another," it causes an imbalance of pressures and disturbs the mind-body. The quality and interaction of the energy winds and *thigle* of the body affect the quality of the flow of the *lungs* in the *tsa* and the movements in the mind-body. In the normal flow of *lung* through the channels, the language basis of consciousness is formed.

Tsa

The *tsa* react in the way that the *lung* in the body react. They are not on their own. They are interdependent with the *lung* and its functions. Yet the major *tsa* have a fixed form that reflects the pattern of the universe. The infinite external universe is represented in our twelve main *tsa* that form at conception. Those *tsa* reflect completely the spacelike quality of our awareness, an essential basis of the wisdom of our buddha-nature. Eventually 72,000 main *tsa*, and related subtle *tsa*, form. The channels of our body are modified according to our projections of the external universe. Our habitual patterning limits the potential of energy channel functioning and results in blockages in the system. Our most subtle channels are always changing according to the activities of our mind. The largest channels, such as the CEC, are fixed in form and are integral to the body's universal functioning.

There are three main or central channels, the CEC and its two "side channels." The CEC is the *trikaya*. The "secret" nature of that and the secret nature of the channel systems must be realized by meditation practice. The blockages in the channels limiting the potential of energy body functioning can be released by meditation practices such as Vase Breathing or by sexual union practice.

Thigle

Thigle is a physical substance, sexual essence, that governs the quality of consciousness and being in the human body. *Thigle* is considered by the *Vajrayana* teachers to be the most precious substance in the human body. The wanton disregard for sexual substances through widespread mindless ejaculation in both sexual engagement with partners and in masturbation is a sign of the general loss of evolutionary quality throughout the species. However, whenever people respect the male and female sexual essences and see them as sacred substances, the health and potential of the human body are safeguarded, and the great potential of the human species in maintained. The greatest triumph of the species, the ability to transform one's body into light (the Rainbow Body of Light), at death or earlier in life, is the result of the knowledge of the light basis of *thigle*. *Vajrayana* masters, such as the Dalai Lama, consider the millions of individual *thigle* to be individual buddhas. They see the waste of *thigle* to be the murder of millions of buddhas and the waste of the light potential of the human form.

In the vision of the *Vajrayana* meditation masters, *thigle* is produced from the finest essence of the digestion of food. That essence in turn is evolved into blood. The blood is filtered (distilled) into the "pure blood of the heart." This creation of blood is seen to take place in the bone marrow, which is in accord with the knowledge of Western science. However, deep insight can see that the blood in the bone marrow, in its highest evolution, is transformed into *thigle*.

Thigle can penetrate bone and unify, in the male, with the seminal fluid in the testes. This is not known to Western science. In women the *thigle* remains closely associated with blood and is called *rhakta*. *Rhakta* is also released in orgasm, but in a much finer form and more as a whole-body emission. Typically in the sexual union practice of *Vajrayana* practitioners, orgasm is withheld; *thigle* is contained, and the light essence of the *thigle* is used to turn awareness to the clear light nature of inherent *rigpa*, luminous clarity. If the *thigle* is released in sexual practice, its light nature is known and it is typically reabsorbed, except for a small amount that is given to the partner as sacred substance to be used for healing or evolution.

Concise Bibliography
of *Vajrayana* Literature in English

Chagdud, Tulku. *Gates to Buddhist Practice.* Junction City, CA: Padma Publishing, 2001.

Chang, G. C. C. *The Six Yogas of Naropa.* Ithaca, NY: Snow Lion Publications, 1963.

Clifford, Terry. *Tibetan Buddhist Medicine and Psychiatry: The Diamond Healing.* New York: Samuel Weiser, Inc., 1984.

Dalai Lama. *A Flash of Lightning in the Dark of Night.* Boston: Shambhala Publications, 1994.

———. *Sleeping, Dreaming, and Dying.* Boston: Wisdom Publications, 1997.

Dowman, Keith. *Sky Dancer: The Secret Life and Songs of the Lady Yeshe Tsogyal.* London: Routledge & Kegan Paul, 1984.

Dudjom Rinpoche. *Counsels from My Heart.* Boston: Shambhala Publications, 2001.

———. *The Nyingma School of Tibetan Buddhism.* London: Wisdom Publications, 1991.

Fremantle, Francesca. *Luminous Emptiness.* Boston: Shambhala Publications, 2001.

——— and Chögyam Trungpa. *The Tibetan Book of the Dead.* Berkeley, CA: Shambhala Publications, 1975.

Gyatrul Rinpoche. *Ancient Wisdom.* Ithaca, NY: Snow Lion Publications, 1993.

Khyentse, Dilgo. *The Heart Treasure of the Enlightened Ones.* Boston: Shambhala Publications, 1992.

Manjusrimitra. *Primordial Experience.* Boston: Shambhala Publications, 1987.

Norbu Rinpoche, Thinley. *White Sail.* Boston: Shambhala Publications, 1992.

Padmasambhava. *Dakini Teachings*. Boston: Shambhala Publications, 1990.

Rangdrol, Tsele Natsok. *The Mirror of Mindfulness*. Boston: Shambhala Publications, 1989.

———. *Natural Liberation*. Boston: Wisdom Publications, 1998.

Reynolds, John. *The Golden Letters*. Ithaca, NY: Snow Lion Publications, 1996.

———. *Self-Liberation Through Seeing with Naked Awareness*. Barrytown, NY: Station Hill Press, 1989.

Sogyal Rinpoche. *The Tibetan Book of Living and Dying*. New York: HarperCollins, 1994.

Thondup Rinpoche, Tulku. *Hidden Teachings of Tibet*. London: Wisdom Publications, 1986.

———. *The Practice of Dzogchen: Writings of Longchen Rabjam*. Ithaca, NY: Snow Lion Publications, 1989.

———. *The Tantric Tradition of the Nyingma*. Marion, MA: Buddhayana, 1984.

Trungpa Rinpoche, Chögyam. *The Collected Works*. Boston: Shambhala Publications, 2004.

Tsogyal, Yeshe. *The Lotus-Born: The Life Story of Padmasambhava*. Boston: Shambhala Publications, 1993.

Glossary

Alaya (Skt.); *kunzhi* (Tib.): Literally it means the basis of all things, the basis of mind and phenomena. Also often called "storehouse consciousness," the basis of all karmic tendencies.

Allopathic medicine: Healing approaches that assume disease and illness are caused by elements outside of the body that have invaded it and must be killed or removed to restore health. Usually used in contrast to homeopathic or naturopathic medicine, which tend to rely on and support the body's internal healing resources.

Ati yoga (Skt.); *Dzogchen* (Tib.): Natural Great Perfection; innate primordial wisdom, free of path or method. Mind-made views and meditations are shattered by free awareness. Disturbing emotions are liberated without any need for reform or remedy. This instruction brings realization not produced from causes. It is instantaneous liberation in wisdom, in the power plenum of absolute space.

Audio-guidance: The use of audio recordings to guide those who listen to facilitate a shift into greater function.

Awareness (Tib. *rigpa*; Skt. *vidya*): When referring to the view of the Great Perfection, "awareness" means self-cognizing consciousness devoid of ignorance and dualistic fixation.

Bardo (Tib.); *antarabhava* (Skt.): The intermediate state. Usually refers to the period between death and the next rebirth. There are also three *bardos* in the present life.

Bindu (Skt.); *thigle* (Tib.): A luminous and brilliant seed syllable. May refer to the point between the eyebrows that connects with the "third eye" *chakra*. See *thigle*.

Bodhicitta (Skt.): "Awakened state of mind." Wisdom heart. (1) The aspiration to attain enlightenment for the sake of all sentient beings. (2) In the context of *Dzogchen*, the innate wakefulness of awakened mind; synonymous with *rigpa*, luminous awareness.

Buddha-nature: The potential for enlightenment or enlightened nature that is inherently present in each sentient being.

Bum Chung (Tib.): Small or Gentle Vase Breathing. It is not *Bum Chen*, Large Vase Breathing, which must be practiced under the close supervision of an accomplished master. Throughout this book the term Vase Breathing refers to Small Vase Breathing, also called "breathing on top of." It may be applied in various medical applications as an awareness-based energy body method.

Chi (Qi): Vital energy. There is external and internal *chi*. "*Chi* is fundamental to Chinese medical thinking, yet no one English word or phrase can adequately capture its meaning. Perhaps we can think of *Chi* as matter on the verge of becoming energy or energy at the point of materializing" (Kaptchuk 1983, 35).

Complementary and Alternative Medicine (CAM): The term for various medical disciplines, mostly traditional, now included in the expanded medical paradigm. Dissatisfaction with conventional medical practices has created great popular interest in and respect for CAM.

Dharmakaya (Skt.); *cho* (Tib.): The first of the three *kayas*, devoid of world but full of extremely powerful energy. It is unmanifest and is inseparable from its form bodies, the *Sambhogakaya* and the *Nirmanakaya*. It is also often used equivalent to *rigpa*.

Dzogchen (Tib.): See *Ati yoga*.

Empowerment (Tib. *wang*): The conferring of power or authorization to practice the *Vajrayana* teachings.

Energy medicine: Medical practices wherein the body is seen to be a body of energy systems and fields; practices of seeing and modifying those fields therapeutically constitutes diagnosis and treatment. Acupuncture, acupressure, bodywork, healing touch, and conscious breathing are each a kind of energy medicine.

Fine breathing: Deep breathing that intentionally absorbs vital energy from the air as well as accessing optimal oxygenation.

Guru Rinpoche (Tib.): "Precious Master," the "Second Buddha" who established *Vajrayana* Buddhism in Tibet in the eighth century. He is also known as Padmasambhava. His compassionate omniscience is with us today in his *terma* (concealed treasures) in *Vajrayana* practice. His methods may enlighten the present and free the future.

Habitual tendencies: Inclinations imprinted in the *alaya* consciousness that can be released by *rigpa*.

Hara (Jap.): The vital center; focal point of *Zen* meditation, comparable to and perhaps the same as the *Tan Tien* in Chinese *Tai Chi* meditation and the Life Vase *(Tse Bum)* in Tibetan *Vajrayana* meditation. It is a receiver for energies breathed into it, for greater function and increase of life force.

Kaya (Skt.); *Ku* (Tib.): Body, simultaneously *Dharmakaya* (unmanifest body), body of light *(Sambhogakaya)*, and flesh and blood of the universe in a form *(Nirmanakaya)*.

Luminosity (Tib. *orsel*): Literally "free from the darkness of unknowing and endowed with the ability to cognize." The two aspects are empty luminosity, like clear open sky, and manifest luminosity, such as five rays of color, images, brilliant spheres of *thigle*. Luminosity is the uncompounded nature present throughout all the world.

Mahayana (Skt.): "The Great Vehicle"; the second major stage in the development of the Buddhist teachings, which emerged in about the first century CE. It distinguished itself from the earlier schools of Buddhism, which it referred to as the *Hinayana*, the "Narrow Path" teachings, a doctrine it viewed as being self-centered. The *Mahayana* is based on the Bodhisattva vow, the unlimited dedication to human service. *Vajrayana* Buddhism is a further development of the *Mahayana*.

Mantra (Skt.): Combinations of seed sound syllables, brilliant *bindu*, radiating healing light from the sound. Almost all mantras start with the radiant *bindu* OM, the crown *chakra*, purifying body into sacred body. *Mantra* also protects the mind. It gives practitioners enlightened sound that resonates healing in the body channels during recitation.

Meditation: A practice that enables people to experience greater levels of awareness and health by shifting consciousness to its essential state, normally blocked by the mind in its undisciplined activity.

Meditation science: The scientific knowledge behind meditation methods from different traditions, with understanding of the short- and long-term effects of the application of those methods. These methods have been tested and proved through centuries of disciplined use, yielding repeatable results in accordance with the scientific method.

Mind-body medicine: An important development in the history of medicine, expanding the medical paradigm in the West since the 1970s, in which meditation and other interventions using the mind enable the body to improve its function. Called self-care in this text, it's seen as the heart of a new medical paradigm.

Mindfulness-Based Stress Reduction (MBSR): The renowned mind-body medicine clinic at the University of Massachusetts Medical Center. Established in 1979, it has trained more than 18,000 people in medicine/meditation methods and has been the model for hundreds of such programs established in the United States, Canada, and Europe.

Nadi (Skt.); *tsa* (Tib.): Energy channel. For full description of the energy channels and their function in accord with *lung* and *thigle*, see the Appendix.

Nectar medicine (Tib. *dutsie;* Skt. *amrita:* the nectar of immortality): A consecrated combination of sacred herbs and blessed substances, energetically endowed with healing power.

Nirmanakaya (Skt.); *tulku* (Tib.): Emanation body. The form *kaya* of the three *kayas*. Form of magical apparition. The aspect of enlightenment that can be perceived by ordinary beings.

Optimal breathing: Breathing practice, such as *Womb Breathing*, in which vital energy from the air and oxygen are breathed.

Padmasambhava: See Guru Rinpoche.

Paradigm: A pattern, example, or model. A concept accepted by most people in an intellectual community, such as the natural sciences.

Paradigm shift: A change in the way individuals or cultures interpret phenomena, a sense of having new eyes or new knowing, leading to new ways of behaving.

Pointing-out instruction (Tib. *mengagde*): The direct instruction given by the teacher so that the disciple recognizes the nature of mind.

Prana (Skt.); *lung* (Tib.): A subtle but powerful life energy pervading all matter; universal life force. Energy currents in the body and in the external universal field. Probably the same as *chi*. Western science refers to it as universal energy and speaks of its field being measurable. It can be breathed and utilized, as in the practice of Vase Breathing.

Reiki (Jap.): A holistic form of natural healing in which universal life force energy flows through the practitioner to the receiver to augment and enhance the natural healing ability inherent within the human body. *Reiki* balances, strengthens, and harmonizes the connection between body, mind, and spirit, promoting a sense of well-being on all levels, for both practitioner and patient.

Sambhogakaya (Skt.); *Long Ku* (Tib.): Between the unmanifest body of the *Dharmakaya* and the manifest body of the *Nirmanakaya* is the semi-manifest body of the *Sambhogakaya*. Referred to as body of bliss, body of communication, it is practiced and experienced as a sacred body of light radiating effectively into the world.

Shamatha (Skt.): Calm Abiding. A meditation practice for calming down and staying calm in order to rest free of the disturbances of the mind. Various concentration techniques are used. The most common is following the breath.

Slow breathing: Deep breathing becomes slow breathing, healthier breathing, using minimal energy. Ancient wisdom says that each life has a certain number of breaths to live, and intentionally slowed breathing brings long life.

Subtle body: Inner body, or energy body. Traditionally, esoteric systems envisioned several bodies inherent in the physical body. Sometimes called astral, mental, and causal bodies, these bodies have been seen to be operating at successively higher frequencies than the physical body. In Buddhist practice the subtle bodies are the *Dharmakaya* and *Sambhogakaya*. They are engaged, activated, and utilized by evolutionary work. Medicine today is more accepting of the presence of an energy body in the physical body, in which subtle body functions are integral to physical functions.

Superknowledge (Skt. *Abhijna*): Powers that naturally arise from meditation, such as those that irreversibly manifested in Shakyamuni Buddha in his enlightenment, and in those who have followed in his path: divine sight; divine hearing; recollection of former lives; cognition of the minds of others; capacity for performing miracles; and in the case of accomplished practitioners, the cognition of the exhaustion of habitual patterns and obscurations.

Tan Tien: Focal point for *Tai Chi* meditation, situated in the navel center. The *Tan Tien* is similar to the Life Vase and the *Hara*, and may be the same.

Tantra: The *Vajrayana* teachings given by the Buddha in his *Sambhogakaya* form. The meaning of the word is "continuity," the innate buddha-nature, which is known as the "*tantra* of the expressed meaning." The general sense of *tantra* is the extraordinary *tantric* scriptures also known as the "*tantra* of the expressing words." Can also refer to the resultant teachings of the *Vajrayana* as a whole.

Terma (Tib.): Treasure. Transmission through concealed treasures, hidden mainly by Guru Rinpoche and Yeshe Tsogyal, to be revealed at the right time by a *terton,* a treasure revealer, for the benefit of all.

Thigle (Tib.); *bindu* (Skt.): A luminous and radiant seed syllable found in the center of each of the *chakras;* also, sperm. See Appendix for detail of function in the energy body.

Trikaya (Skt.): *Dharmakaya, Sambhogakaya,* and *Nirmanakaya.* The three *kayas* as ground are essence, nature, and expression; as path they are bliss, clarity, and nonthought; and as fruition they are the three *kayas* of Buddhahood.

Vajra (Skt.); *dorje* (Tib.): "Diamond," "king of stones." As an adjective it means "indestructible," "invincible," or "firm." The ultimate *vajra* is emptiness, complete openness; the conventional *vajra* is the ritual implement, mostly cast metal.

Vajrayana: The Diamond Vehicle; the Buddhism of Tibet; the ultimate stage of the development of the Buddha's teachings. Based on the vow of compassionate service to all life, *Vajrayana* Buddhism is known for its variety of profound methods.

Vase Breathing: This practice, a treasure of ancient wisdom, is characterized by breathing vital essence from the air down into the Life Vase, *Tse Bum* (Tib.), in the navel center, which feeds the energy up into the central psychic channel for greater function.

Vipashyana (Skt.): Clear or wider seeing; panoramic awareness; extraordinary insight; "Wisdom Mind" arising from *Shamatha* practice. Also a psychological basis of Vase Breathing.

Visualization: Most often a concentration method in which the whole body, a specific body system, or body process is envisioned purposefully, to alter the body's biology beneficially. To be most successful visualization should be based on calming meditation. In practices such as Vase Breathing, the energy body and its systems are visualized to access their potential.

Yoga: Literally "union." Originally a general category for various kinds of meditation practice, today in the West *yoga* usually refers to *hatha yoga*, stretching and breathing exercises, which can be beneficial in prenatal care. Tibetan *yoga* practice is based on Vase Breathing and a progressive development of the realization and utilization of the potential of the energy body.

Index

12 Steps, 262, 263, 326, 368

A

AA, 264, 267, 269
Abhijna, 347
acne, 18
acupressure, 121, 132, 148, 344
acupuncture, xv, 22, 109, 113, 117,
   121, 148, 149, 344
addiction, xiv, xv, 14, 262, 268
adrenal glands, 67, 278
AIDS, 6, 21, 41, 50, 52, 54, 67, 152,
   153, 154, 208, 367
alaya, 92, 344
alpha state, 16
alpha wave, 16, 17, 47
Alzheimer's, xviii, 154, 289, 290, 291,
   292, 333, 367
Alzheimer's care, xviii, 333
anatomy, 6, 11, 13, 103, 114, 194,
   231
anxiety, xiv, 23, 52, 53, 54, 55, 56, 60,
   64, 65, 66, 69, 71, 72, 73, 74, 76, 88,
   91, 152, 168, 202, 228, 283, 330
arthritis, 18, 154
assumptions, 8, 32, 83, 100, 143, 144
asthma, 14, 70, 280
astral, 95, 108, 109, 347
Atman, 33, 137
ASC (altered state of consciousness),
   84
audio-guidance, 18, 160, 170, 223,
   233, 234, 241, 246, 292, 298, 304

audio-guide, 155, 175, 176, 220, 223,
   233, 234, 241, 246, 289, 291, 292,
   297, 298, 301, 302, 304
autism, 290
awareness, xvi, 3, 4, 16, 17, 25, 26,
   33, 36, 37, 42, 43, 45, 47, 50, 52, 53,
   54, 58, 59, 60, 61, 62, 63, 64, 66, 69,
   74, 83, 85, 87, 88, 92, 93, 95, 97, 98,
   99, 106, 109, 110, 111, 112, 113,
   114, 117, 124, 137, 146, 151, 155,
   166, 167, 168, 169, 171, 172, 175,
   181, 182, 185, 188, 189, 190, 191,
   193, 194, 195, 196, 198, 200, 201,
   203, 204, 205, 206, 212, 215, 230,
   237, 238, 239, 242, 243, 244, 251,
   254, 258, 270, 289, 290, 291, 297,
   301, 302, 312, 315, 333, 336, 337,
   338, 342, 343, 345, 349
   pure awareness, 97
Ayurveda, 35, 36, 37

B

balance, 12, 23, 27, 53, 62, 65, 66, 67,
   100, 111, 136, 149, 159, 195, 235,
   289, 333
bedwetting, 16
behavioral shifts, 70
belief, 10, 12, 28, 48, 86, 95, 262,
   330
beliefs, 8, 85, 93, 100, 106, 146
BF, 14, 15, 16
Bible, 4, 27, 28, 325
bindu, 113, 114, 345, 348

biofeedback, 14, 15, 16, 75, 166, 169, 171, 172
Biofeedback Research Society, 13
biophysics, xviii, 6
bliss technique, 36
blood flow, 71, 72, 76, 181, 182, 227, 271, 282
blood pressure, 13, 14, 19, 49, 54, 58, 67, 71, 76, 99, 165, 170, 281
blood-oxygen, 13
blood-pressure, 13
Bodhicitta, 153, 343
body of light, 344, 347
Boston, 30, 51
Brahman, 3, 137
brain, 13, 15, 16, 17, 21, 35, 46, 47, 49, 53, 66, 67, 68, 83, 85, 86, 87, 89, 116, 117, 128, 150, 154, 165, 167, 266, 279, 290, 291
brain-wave, 13, 16, 46, 47, 49, 86, 128
breathing, 34, 42, 48, 50, 52, 53, 58, 60, 62, 69, 113, 117, 122, 123, 124, 138, 151, 152, 185, 186, 187, 193, 194, 195, 196, 198, 199, 200, 201, 202, 203, 205, 210, 231, 232, 234, 235, 236, 237, 238, 239, 242, 243, 245, 279, 280, 281, 293, 311, 312, 330, 335, 343, 344, 347, 348, 349
buddha-nature, 113, 258, 337, 348
Buddhist, 3, 27, 37, 38, 39, 40, 41, 47, 49, 50, 51, 59, 92, 97, 109, 110, 111, 112, 113, 114, 124, 125, 126, 134, 150, 207, 218, 270, 272, 301, 319, 335, 340, 347, 365
Bum Chung, 42, 43, 117, 195, 343
burns, 18, 64, 196, 259, 267

C
Calm Birth, 220, 221, 252, 336, 365, 366, 367, 368, 369
cancer, xviii, 7, 17, 18, 21, 36, 52, 53, 54, 66, 67, 70, 72, 73, 74, 152, 207, 208, 367
cancer care, xviii, 74, 152, 207, 367
cardiac arrhythmia, 14, 55, 71
cardiovascular care, xviii, 73, 367
cardiovascular disease, 70
caregiver, 146, 155, 289, 291, 301
Cartesian split, 4
causal body, 108, 109, 111, 137, 148, 154, 347
cell, 8, 9, 28, 66, 120, 127, 131, 132, 187
cells, 6, 7, 8, 17, 21, 35, 66, 67, 99, 113, 125, 131, 132, 136, 159, 165, 166, 179, 186, 225, 251, 281, 300, 313, 320, 321
central channel, 117, 2935, 236
ceremony, 256, 259
chakra, 66, 114, 115, 117, 139, 194, 195, 198, 232, 336, 342, 345, 348
chemistry, 6, 90, 290
chemotherapy, 14, 54
chi, 67, 122, 123, 124, 126, 148, 193, 194, 232, 236, 237, 335, 336, 343, 346
Chi Gung, 22
child, 221, 222, 228, 229, 238, 239, 240, 242, 243, 244, 245, 247, 249, 250, 251, 272, 330
childbirth, xviii, 40, 152, 154, 219, 220, 221, 231, 245, 247, 330, 333, 366, 367
children, 13, 15, 17, 239, 240, 265, 367, 368

China, 21, 22, 37
Christ Consciousness, 105, 137
Christian, 27, 29, 30, 31, 32, 105, 106,
    125, 269, 312
Christian Science, 30, 262
Christianity, 27, 37, 96, 104, 105
chronic conditions, 70, 150
Church, 4, 28, 30, 31, 105, 262
coma, 154, 297, 312
comatose, 154, 155, 212, 289, 290,
    291, 301, 302, 333
community, 6, 20, 27, 29, 57, 83, 145,
    157, 261, 324, 346
Compassionate Breathing, 1, 42, 43,
    152, 154, 159, 207, 210, 211, 212,
    215, 216, 218, 247, 249, 251, 286
Complementary and Alternative
    Medicine, xv, 343
CAM, xv, xviii, 15, 343
complications, 11, 75, 76, 152
computer games, 15
concentration, 15, 34, 60, 63, 89, 90,
    176, 268, 269, 281, 347, 349
connective tissue matrix, 132
conscious breathing, 344
consciousness, 3, 4, 6, 7, 9, 17, 18, 20,
    26, 29, 33, 36, 45, 51, 56, 57, 83, 84,
    85, 86, 87, 88, 89, 90, 91, 92, 94, 95,
    96, 99, 100, 104, 105, 109, 110, 114,
    125, 128, 130, 131, 146, 154, 155,
    159, 166, 176, 253, 254, 265, 266,
    274, 282, 286, 311, 312, 314, 315,
    321, 322, 324, 325, 326, 327, 329,
    330, 333, 337, 338, 342, 344, 345,
    367, 368
altered state of consciousness
    [ASC], 84
discrete states, 86

constipation, 14
convalescence, 151
coronary care, 152
crystal, 22, 23, 132, 148, 149
cultures, xv, xviii, 3, 20, 22, 25, 26,
    37, 43, 45, 56, 114, 121, 125, 130,
    145, 253, 262, 312, 317, 326, 346
cybernetics, xviii, 6, 20, 89, 367
cycles, 10, 128

D
Dalai Lama, 50, 338, 340, 365
death, xiv, xv, xviii, 30, 40, 46, 70, 73,
    74, 76, 92, 107, 125, 152, 153, 154,
    155, 160, 190, 204, 212, 214, 215,
    245, 258, 290, 299, 300, 301, 302,
    305, 306, 330, 332, 338, 342
deep breathing, 344, 347
dementia, 290
depression, 54, 64, 71, 74, 152
Dharmakaya, 93, 110, 111, 112, 113,
    124, 137, 139, 148, 154, 319, 336,
    343, 344, 347, 348
DHEA, 65, 67, 68
diabetes, 18, 52, 67, 76
digestive disorders, 14
diseases, xiv, 52, 65, 75, 151
doctor, xiv, xv, xvii, 7, 9, 10, 37, 38,
    39, 40, 46, 116, 144, 146, 153, 175,
    245, 278, 284, 290, 312, 330, 331,
    335, 367
drug protocols, xv
drug reactions, xiv, 70, 76
drugs, xiv, 10, 64, 84, 87, 221, 232,
    247, 301, 332

E
eczema, 18

education, xvii, xviii, 76, 329, 330, 331
EEG, 16, 55, 126, 141, 279, 287
ego, 20, 88, 98
electrocardiograms
  EKG, 120
electroencephalogram
  EEG, 126
electromagnetic signature, 8
electromagnetics, xviii
emanation body, 346
emotions, 6, 8, 11, 25, 60, 83, 87, 96, 100, 108, 109, 111, 112, 130, 143, 157, 165, 166, 204, 222, 254, 275, 278, 318, 324, 342
Empowerment, 69, 343
emptiness, 110, 111, 113, 348
endocrine system, 115
endorphins, 64, 65, 67, 68, 281
energy body, 43, 137, 159, 220, 231, 267, 347
energy channel, 346
energy fields, 136, 137, 144
Energy medicine, 344
enlightenment, 56, 343, 346, 347
epilepsy, 14
equilibrium, 143, 144
Era I, xvi, xvii, 12, 103, 140, 149, 154, 157, 165, 290, 301, 303, 311
Era II, xvii, xviii, xix, 103, 140, 149, 332, 333
Era III, xvii, xviii, xix, 140, 149, 157, 160, 301, 332, 333
esoteric, 89, 318, 347
estrogen, 8
etheric, 107, 108, 109, 137
etheric body, 108
exercise, 59, 150

experiments, 11, 13, 14, 16, 23, 118, 130, 312, 318

F
family, 29, 89, 130, 144, 146, 157, 228, 238, 239, 281, 285, 319
father, 240, 242, 290, 336
fatigue, 151
feedback, 13, 15, 22, 128, 133, 134
field, xiv, xviii, xix, 13, 19, 20, 21, 39, 58, 63, 84, 103, 107, 108, 110, 117, 118, 119, 120, 121, 122, 123, 124, 125, 126, 127, 128, 129, 130, 131, 135, 136, 137, 144, 147, 148, 149, 154, 158, 159, 165, 166, 173, 174, 183, 188, 194, 198, 217, 218, 219, 231, 232, 237, 239, 240, 251, 253, 254, 256, 258, 259, 260, 270, 280, 300, 303, 318, 319, 320, 321, 322, 323, 326, 333, 335, 336, 344, 346, 368
  biomagnetic, 119
  morphogenetic, 129
films, 278
frequencies, 109, 119, 125, 127, 128, 347
friends, 20, 144, 146, 157, 281, 285

G
give birth, xviii
Global Consciousness Project, 323, 325
goiter, 151
group, xix, 11, 20, 30, 72, 83, 145, 173, 368
group healing, xix
guided meditation, 59, 90, 155, 289
Guru Rinpoche, 344, 346, 348

H

Habitual tendencies, 344

Hara, 193, 344, 348

Harvard, xvii, 47, 48, 51, 53, 55, 129, 173

hatha yoga, 349

headache, 14, 18, 70, 150

healer, 11, 21, 29, 30, 38, 77, 146, 156, 158, 209, 211, 215, 218, 319

healers, xv, 23, 26, 100, 132, 147, 158, 262, 312

healing touch, 148, 344

health, xiv, xv, xvii, xix, 9, 13, 14, 31, 41, 42, 43, 48, 50, 51, 52, 53, 59, 64, 65, 67, 68, 69, 70, 76, 77, 98, 111, 126, 145, 147, 149, 154, 157, 158, 160, 165, 172, 176, 193, 195, 200, 206, 221, 247, 250, 253, 281, 282, 289, 329, 330, 331, 332, 333, 338, 342, 345, 366, 368

health care, xv, xvii

heart conditions, 59

heart disease, 52, 57, 59, 70, 71, 72, 73

heart disorders, 151

Higher Self, 109, 137, 270

Hindu, 3, 27, 33, 37, 50, 55, 92, 93, 113, 114, 123, 319, 322, 325, 335

holistic health, xvi

homeopathy, xv, 22

hospital care, xiv, 70, 146

hot flashes, 14

hypertension, 14, 54, 72, 151, 174, 280

hypometabolic state, 48

hypothalamus, 115, 116

I

Illness, 1, 9, 24, 99, 100, 140, 160, 277, 282, 286, 311, 312, 313, 314, 315

imagery, 9, 16, 17, 18, 19, 22, 84, 143, 145, 146, 149, 150, 159, 160, 171, 195, 268

Imagery, 16, 18, 23, 78, 150, 160

imagination, 17, 18, 108, 268

immune enhancement, 152

immune system, 10, 65, 66, 67, 195, 209, 245, 281, 333

incontinence, 14

India, 32, 35, 37, 38, 45, 59, 66, 95, 321

Institute of Noetic Sciences, xviii

intention, xv, xix, 17, 21, 111, 145, 146, 147, 148, 149, 153, 195, 210, 214, 238, 251, 256, 258, 259, 266, 271, 333

internal environment, 18

Islam, 37, 96, 104

J

Jewish, 27, 29

joke, 281, 283, 285, 286

Judaism, 29, 96, 104, 105

Judeo-Christian, 30

K

karma, 33, 92, 93, 256, 258, 260

kayas, 343, 346, 348

Kriya Yoga, 35, 101, 141

L

laughter, 278, 279, 280, 281, 282

laying on of hands, 11, 23, 27, 148, 368

Leprosy, 153

life force, 62, 104, 121, 122, 123, 124,
148, 154, 175, 176, 190, 195, 200,
209, 224, 225, 227, 228, 299, 336,
344, 346
light, 9, 32, 35, 49, 50, 86, 95, 103,
110, 111, 112, 119, 120, 125, 126,
128, 133, 136, 137, 138, 139, 147,
153, 158, 176, 186, 187, 194, 196,
198, 199, 203, 205, 209, 210, 211,
212, 214, 215, 216, 222, 245, 248,
249, 250, 251, 254, 258, 259, 267,
294, 299, 300, 302, 305, 336, 338,
339, 344
living systems, 313
luminosity, 344
lung, 74, 123, 124, 335, 336, 337, 345,
346

M
magnetosphere, 127
Maharishi Effect, 57, 325, 327
mantra, 56, 57, 69, 96, 258, 344,
345
matter, 3, 108, 130, 278
Matter, 321
maya, 3
Mayo Clinic, 14, 15
medical arts, xv
medical establishment, xiv, xvii, 22,
214, 220, 365
medical intuitives, 144
medical paradigm, xv, xvi, 42, 77,
103, 329, 331, 343, 345
medical practice, xix
medical protocol, 12
medical science, xiv, 64, 103
medicine, xiv, xv, xvi, xvii, xviii, xix,
9, 10, 12, 16, 18, 21, 38, 39, 40, 45,
47, 48, 51, 63, 67, 68, 69, 75, 77,
103, 113, 132, 140, 144, 145, 149,
152, 153, 154, 157, 158, 160, 165,
173, 174, 175, 176, 198, 200, 201,
205, 207, 217, 218, 219, 221, 245,
277, 279, 281, 290, 301, 303, 311,
312, 317, 330, 331, 332, 333, 335,
342, 344, 345, 365, 366, 367
allopathic, xv, 77, 144
alternative medicine, xvi
Ayurvedic medicine, 39, 335
field of, xiv
new medicine, xix
preventive, 151
scientific, xiv, xv, xvi, xvii, 7, 8, 12,
20, 21, 23, 29, 35, 39, 77, 84, 85,
103, 117, 129, 140, 143, 207, 312,
345
transpersonal, 145
mediere, 68
meditation science, xv, xviii, 43, 97,
114, 115, 123, 124, 219, 232, 235,
367
melatonin, 53, 65, 66, 67, 73
memory loss, 290
mental, 12, 26, 34, 49, 56, 58, 84, 89,
90, 94, 95, 99, 108, 109, 143, 155,
168, 179, 215, 216, 253, 254, 290,
291, 302, 305
mental body, 108, 347
metaphysical, 105
mice, 11
migraine, 14, 18, 70
Mind/Body Clinic, 48, 51, 53, 54
mind-body, 45, 97, 100, 112, 136, 137,
150, 153, 159, 253, 280
mind-body medicine, 45, 345
mind-body methods, xvii

mindfulness, 42, 50, 51, 53, 59, 60, 61, 62, 64, 151, 152, 175, 194, 196, 221, 231

mindfulness meditation, 42, 51, 61, 62, 64, 152, 175, 194, 196, 221, 231

Mindfulness-Based Stress Reduction (MBSR), 51, 345

miracles, 29, 105, 187, 299, 300, 347

model, xiv, xvi, xvii, xviii, xix, 7, 19, 23, 29, 51, 52, 84, 85, 86, 88, 89, 92, 93, 103, 104, 105, 106, 108, 109, 111, 112, 113, 114, 115, 122, 130, 132, 135, 136, 137, 140, 143, 144, 147, 148, 149, 156, 157, 158, 159, 167, 231, 313, 315, 317, 318, 319, 321, 326, 335, 345, 346, 365, 366

mood, 67, 89, 319

Morphic Resonance, 129, 131, 320

mother, 28, 208, 209, 240, 245, 290, 336

multi-body, 104

multifold body, 108

Mundaka Upanishad, 3

muscles, 67, 119, 189, 226, 227

Muslim, 27, 38, 105

mystical experience, 16

N

nadi, 113, 116, 117, 123, 132, 345

National Institutes of Health, xv, 8, 21

nausea and vomiting, 14, 54

near-death care, xviii

near-death states, 301

nerve force, 123

nerves, 62, 116, 117, 123, 127, 176, 180, 181, 182, 183, 184, 185, 186, 187, 201, 221, 224, 226, 227, 228, 266

neuropeptides, 8

New Testament, 105, 325

New Thought, 30, 31, 32, 105, 106, 158, 255, 262, 270, 271, 312, 325, 368

newborn, 240

Nirmanakaya, 110, 111, 112, 137, 148, 154, 343, 344, 346, 348

nirvana, 92, 96

nonlocal mind, 297

nonlocality, 322, 324

nurse, xv, 12, 367

Nyingma, 50, 340, 341, 365

O

om, 258

om ah hung, 258

openness, 112, 158, 211, 348

Oversoul, 106, 137

oxygen, 35, 46, 49, 58, 122, 194, 231, 237, 279, 280, 346

oxygenation, 76, 196, 344

P

Padmasambhava, 38, 41, 44, 303, 340, 341, 344, 346

Padre Pio, 28

pain, xiv, xvi, 12, 17, 18, 19, 28, 33, 36, 52, 53, 54, 60, 62, 64, 65, 66, 68, 71, 76, 85, 86, 111, 145, 150, 152, 178, 179, 180, 184, 185, 198, 204, 205, 225, 245, 269, 278, 279, 311

paradigm, xiv, xviii, 16, 37, 73, 103, 174, 220, 312, 317, 318, 366, 368

paradigm shift, xiv, xvi, 346, 366

patients, xv, xvi, 13, 17, 18, 19, 21, 30,

51, 53, 58, 74, 75, 144, 145, 146,
152, 154, 155, 156, 174, 175, 208,
217, 278, 279, 281, 290
patterns of vibration, 118
Pentecostal, 28, 105
perception, 4, 29, 34, 85, 96, 106, 165,
166, 203, 318, 366
pharmaceutical, xiv, xv, 332
pharmaceuticals, 8, 156
physical body, 108, 113
physics, 6, 84, 90, 121, 131
pineal gland, 53, 66, 115
placebo, 9, 10, 21
plants, 11, 40, 122, 129, 313
PMS (premenstrual syndrome), 14
postnatal care, 220, 221, 222, 231,
232, 330
postoperative conditions, 151
posture, 61, 62, 133, 168
power, xvii, xix, 4, 6, 7, 17, 19, 23, 32,
38, 45, 53, 58, 77, 111, 114, 115,
122, 125, 145, 148, 154, 168, 169,
185, 187, 194, 195, 198, 211, 229,
232, 234, 235, 238, 240, 243, 251,
256, 258, 262, 270, 274, 330, 332,
342, 343, 345
Practice of Healing, 221, 245, 246
prana, 33, 34, 58, 113, 114, 117, 122,
123, 124, 148, 194, 232, 236, 237,
335, 336, 346
prayer, 27, 28, 31, 48, 105, 146, 147,
159, 160, 260, 272, 325, 326
Precious Master, 344
pregnancy, 9
prenatal care, 220, 231, 330, 349
prescription, xiv, 10, 333
progressive neuromuscular release,
96, 150, 221, 222

Progressive Relaxation, 61, 78, 145,
150, 151, 160, 173, 176, 192, 221,
252, 268, 330
psychiatry, 84, 253
psycho-emotional illness, xiv
psychology, 6, 20, 37, 38, 83, 84, 86,
88, 89, 90, 104, 253
transpersonal, 19
psychoneuroimmunology, 6, 368
puja, 256
pun, 281, 283, 284

Q
Qabalah, 29, 44
Quantum mechanics, 322
quantum physics, xviii, 6, 7, 254,
320

R
radiation, 10, 73
random number generators, 323
Raynaud's disease, 14
reality, 3, 4, 7, 52, 85, 86, 94, 96, 98,
101, 106, 121, 137, 168, 211, 254,
282, 302
receptors, 8, 127, 132
recovery, 9, 68, 146, 155, 268, 277,
279
reflexology, 148
Reiki, 12, 13, 147, 148, 159, 346, 368
Relaxation Response, 48, 53, 78, 146
release, xix, 23, 31, 97, 99, 138, 139,
155, 173, 178, 179, 180, 182, 187,
188, 191, 194, 212, 220-230, 254,
259, 260, 273, 275, 281, 282, 283,
285, 297, 301, 302, 312, 326
religion, 4, 6, 59, 106, 107
resonant pattern, 23, 131, 135

reverse, 7, 17, 49, 56, 71, 174, 216, 245, 284, 290, 302, 323

rigpa, 92, 93, 96, 98, 99, 137, 194, 270, 315, 339, 342, 343, 344

Riwo Sang Cho, 256, 259

S

samadhi, 33, 96

Sambhogakaya, 110, 111, 112, 137, 147, 319, 343, 344, 347, 348

sang, 256, 259, 260

Sanskrit, 3, 33, 51, 56, 58, 92, 93, 94, 98, 110, 113, 115, 116

satori, 69

satsang, 319

Schumann's Resonances, 127

science, xvi, xviii, 4, 6, 16, 32, 35, 41, 46, 47, 48, 49, 50, 59, 77, 104, 107, 122, 124, 131, 139, 268, 312, 318, 331, 335, 338, 345, 346, 366, 367

scientific literature, 11

scientific medicine, xiv, xvii, 21, 140, 143, 312

scientists, 4, 45, 104

self-care, xvii, xviii, 43, 54, 174, 175, 176, 221, 289, 329, 330, 331, 332, 333

self-organization, 134

September 11, 2001, 323, 325

serotonin, 65, 67

shaman, 3, 4, 23, 25, 121, 254, 267

shamanic practices, 20, 26, 96

shamanic traditions, 22, 23, 25, 26, 121, 157, 254, 272, 312

Shamatha, 42, 59, 61, 347, 349

sickness, 60, 147, 152, 208, 209, 210, 212, 214, 215, 216, 217, 218, 245, 248

sitting, 46, 47, 49, 52, 53, 56, 60, 61, 62, 174, 196, 198, 220, 231, 234, 268, 269, 323

skin, 13, 47, 49, 55, 86, 104, 317, 318

sleep, 14, 55, 58, 67, 69, 95, 100, 112, 128, 151, 196, 203, 222, 238, 278, 312

sleep disorders, 14

Slow breathing, 347

small self, 98

somatic processes, 9

soul, 3, 26, 29, 95, 104, 106, 108, 123, 254

spasm, 151

spine, 61, 62, 187, 198, 229, 235, 277

spirit, 3, 4, 6, 19, 20, 58, 106, 107, 108, 109, 111, 113, 123, 147, 157, 209, 277, 279, 285, 286, 317, 346

Spirit, 27, 29, 44, 105, 106, 114, 137, 141, 144, 160, 334

spiritual traditions, 19, 271, 325

stress-busters, 65

stroke, 57, 70, 71

studies, 9, 12, 13, 15, 16, 19, 20, 21, 25, 45, 47, 55, 56, 57, 74, 146, 207, 279, 281, 367

subconscious, 8, 92, 93, 130, 158, 268

subtle body, 108, 347

suffering, 19, 60, 64, 147, 152, 153, 154, 179, 180, 205, 208, 209, 210, 211, 212, 214, 215, 216, 217, 218, 248, 249, 250, 251, 253, 261, 280, 281, 283, 286, 315, 326

Sufi, 27, 89

surgery, xiv, xvii, 40, 55, 70, 75, 146, 152, 211, 221, 228, 247, 332

surgical technology, xiv

symbols, 17, 18, 145

symptoms, xvii, 9, 10, 11, 17, 22, 23, 49, 52, 54, 60, 68, 69, 76, 100, 150, 155, 174, 275, 282, 290, 311, 312, 315, 333
system, 6, 8, 37, 39, 42, 65, 75, 84, 112, 115, 116, 117, 121, 122, 133, 134, 135, 144, 157, 166, 167, 179, 180, 185, 187, 191, 194, 195, 202, 218, 222, 225, 227, 235, 264, 319, 320, 335, 337, 344, 347, 349, 367
    living systems, 134

T
Tai Chi, 22, 193, 344, 348
Tan Tien, 193, 199, 344, 348
Therapeutic Touch, 12, 24, 148
thigle, 114, 335, 336, 337, 338, 339, 342, 344, 346, 348
thought, 4, 8, 9, 13, 16, 23, 26, 29, 32, 56, 58, 66, 69, 75, 83, 87, 89, 96, 98, 106, 108, 136, 139, 143, 150, 158, 201, 203, 204, 237, 262, 265, 266, 269, 271, 273, 278, 282, 301, 313, 318, 322
Tibet, 37, 38, 39, 40, 41, 121, 153, 231, 303, 341, 344, 348
Tibetan medicine, 40
TM, 50, 55, 56, 57, 58, 69
Tong Len, 42, 43, 153, 207, 301, 365
training programs, xix, 331
trance, 28, 97, 204
trance states, 17, 26
Transcendental Meditation, 50, 55, 57, 79, 326
Transcendentalist, 106
transformation, xix, 101, 303, 312, 330

Transformative Compassionate Breathing, 245
transpersonal medicine, xvii, 157
trikaya, 109, 110, 112, 137, 326, 337, 348
tsa, 335, 336, 337, 346
Tse Bum, 124, 193, 344, 349
TT, 12, 13
tuberculosis, 151
turiya, 95, 96
twentieth century, xiv, 6, 22, 28, 30, 37, 89, 133

U
ulcer, 151
UMMC, 51, 52, 53, 58, 59, 61, 63, 64, 66, 70, 73, 175, 195, 221
unconscious, 20, 62, 92, 93, 180, 188, 189, 190, 196, 230, 238, 267, 301
Universal Energy Field, 124
University of Massachusetts Medical Center, 221, 345
UMMC, 51
Upanishads, 93, 113, 114, 122

V
Vajrayana, 1, 41, 47, 59, 123, 193, 199, 231, 256, 260, 303, 326, 335, 338, 340, 343, 344, 348
Vase Breathing, 42, 43, 117, 151, 152, 159, 193, 194, 195, 196, 201, 203, 204, 205, 337, 343, 346, 348, 349, 365
Vedas, 33, 66, 93, 115
Vedic traditions, 3, 33
vibration, 119, 120, 125, 147
video, 15, 281
vidya, 98, 342

Vipashyana, 42, 43, 50, 59, 61, 69, 151, 196, 349, 365

visualization, 11, 16, 24, 145, 231, 349

W

water, 11, 28, 119, 127, 132, 166, 264, 267

wave-form, 118, 132, 159, 318, 322

wavicles, 125, 270, 321, 322

web of life, 317

What the BLEEP Do We Know!?, 8, 118, 322

wisdom, xviii, 20, 29, 38, 43, 84, 92, 111, 122, 125, 195, 200, 211, 212, 219, 235, 258, 260, 293, 305, 306, 307, 313, 319, 337, 342, 347, 349

witches, 26, 325

Womb Breathing, 231

World War II, xiv, 28

Y

Yeshe Tsogyal, 39, 41, 340, 341, 348

yoga, 33, 34, 35, 37, 45, 53, 89, 94, 95, 122, 123, 173, 224, 326, 335, 342, 343, 349

yogi, 32, 35, 46, 47, 92, 93, 313

Z

Zen, 16, 46, 47, 50, 59, 69, 79, 126, 141, 193, 344

zungwa, 98

Acknowledgments

THIS BOOK PROBABLY would not have been completed if it weren't for the interest of Richard Grossinger, publisher of North Atlantic Books. Robert told Richard about the unfinished *Calm Healing* manuscript just after concluding the *Calm Birth* book. It was Richard's interest that encouraged Robert to ask Ruth to partner with him in the project. Richard's support is not simply that of a businessman engaged in publishing. He has published several important books concerned with medicine, including *Planet Medicine*, an encyclopedic work engaging the origins and modalities of the many approaches to medicine and healing. Richard's support for the *Calm Healing* project has been that of a silent partner in the work nurturing the project.

We also would like to express our deep appreciation to all the writers and publishers who gave us permission to include their words in our attempt to clarify and further develop an emerging model of the human mind-body.

Robert's Acknowledgments

Most important for me as an inspiration for this book is H. H. Dudjom Rinpoche, former head of the Nyingma Lineage of Tibetan Buddhism and Dzogchen lama of the Dalai Lama. His personal guidance and teachings on the nature of mind and body are my greatest resource. His son and lineage heir, H. H. Shenphen Rinpoche, was my personal lama and trainer for the Vase Breathing and visualization-based methods presented in this book. The teachings, transmissions, and empowerments of Dudjom Rinpoche and Shenphen Rinpoche have remained a special source of life and grace for me in my work in the medical establishment. I'll be forever grateful.

The meditation master Chögyam Trungpa Rinpoche, my first lama, with whom I worked from 1970 to 1980, inspired me to practice *Vipashyana* and *Tong Len* meditation with all my heart for ten years and was a great model for how to teach Buddhist psychological methods in the West.

The development of the MediGrace program was enabled by Gerald Lehrburger, MD, director of the Health Research Institute, Ashland, Oregon. His support and guidance have been a major factor in the progress of the program that is the basis of this book. He was the first member of the MediGrace board of directors and remains a continuing advisor and advocate.

Early in the emergence of MediGrace I began to write a book to describe the paradigm shift in medicine that encouraged new kinds of health care and to publish the methods. But after I had made a draft of the book *Calm Healing*, I became absorbed in the childbirth meditation work and writing the book presenting that program: *Calm Birth: New Method for Conscious Childbirth* (North Atlantic Books 2005). I suspended the work on the *Calm Healing* book. Then, early in 2005, I met Dr. Ruth Miller, who accepted my offer to be partners in the completion of the *Calm Healing* book. Ruth is an exceptional teacher of mind-body science and an accomplished writer. Her skills in language and research, her knowledge of science and healing methods, were just what the *Calm Healing* project needed to come to fruition. The book wouldn't exist without her, and with her participation it became much more than it would have been had I been able to complete it alone.

Ruth's Acknowledgments

As always happens when completing a project like this, far more people contribute to the effort than one can properly acknowledge. So, to all those who allowed their lives and schedules to be disrupted by the time I spent working on this project, please accept my deep gratitude and appreciation—especially Con and Ayama.

Acknowledgments

Special thanks are also owed to O. W. Markley, former instructor and mentor, and longtime friend, for his assistance in the early development of the model from which I have been working and for his continuing supply of useful and informative resources as the model evolves. To Robert, whose perception that what I might bring to this project would be useful and whose willingness to let my vision build on his own created an opening for something entirely new, deep appreciation. It was worth it.

About the Authors

Robert Bruce Newman is the Executive Director of MediGrace, Inc. and developed most of the methods described in this text. Instead of going to medical school, Mr. Newman chose to venture into what turned out to be a twenty-year apprenticeship with Tibetan meditation masters and doctors. In 1991, with Drs. John Sutton and Craig Spaniol of NASA, he founded MediGrace as a nonprofit organization dedicated to extend the use of meditation science and mind-body science in medicine. Now located in Southern Oregon, with the continuing help of various medical professionals Mr. Newman has presented more than eighty training seminars in West Coast hospitals since 1997, all with the support of the California Board of Registered Nursing. He has developed programs and methods for cancer care, cardiovascular care, HIV/AIDS care, and Alzheimer's care. Health care providers, such as Asante, the major owner-operator of hospitals in Southern Oregon, that had found that their own medical professionals, doctors and nurses, suffered from various stress-related conditions, paid for their providers to take the medicine/meditation programs Mr. Newman offered in their hospitals.

In 1998 he initiated a program in childbirth meditation, Calm Birth, which has been receiving international support. His book *Calm Birth: New Method for Conscious Childbirth* was published by North Atlantic Books in 2005.

He has taught at the University of Colorado, Naropa University, and the City University of New York.

Ruth L. Miller, Ph.D., has devoted her life to the understanding of consciousness and our human capacity to create. While married and raising children, she attended ten colleges, acquiring four degrees (in anthropology, environmental studies, cybernetics, and systems science) and earned a living as a consulting futurist and college professor—all with the purpose of discovering and facilitating the true nature of human consciousness. When the inevitable physical and emotional collapse came, she immersed herself in the fields of psychoneuroimmunology and metaphysics, becoming a *Reiki* practitioner as a way to understand the "laying on of hands." Through offering *Reiki* to self and others, along with various forms of meditation and the *12 Steps to Freedom* practice, she restored her body to full health and function. After a divorce and when the children were grown, she completed studying for the ministry and was ordained as a New Thought minister. As such, she has worked as a "circuit riding preacher" across the state of Oregon, giving Sunday talks and programs and offering workshops and classes on metaphysics, social consciousness, and the potential of the emerging paradigm. Working with other like-minded folks, Ruth has helped found numerous service and spiritual organizations in Oregon, including New West Seminary in Oregon City, the Unitarian Universalist Fellowship and its offspring, a Fair Trade shop called the Creative Alternative in Grants Pass, WiseWoman Press in Beaverton, and The Wisdom Centers of Oregon. She has written a number of books, including *150 Years of Healing: The Lives and Works of America's Great New Thought Healers; An Uncommon Book of Prayer;* and *Unveiling Your Hidden Power: Emma Curtis Hopkins' Metaphysics for the 21st Century.* She continues to seek greater understanding of the nature of human consciousness and works with individuals and groups to expand experience of the human potential.

A graduate of Amherst College, **Richard Grossinger** received a Ph.D. in anthropology from the University of Michigan. He is the author of many books, including *Planet Medicine; The Night Sky; Embryogenesis: Species, Gender, and Identity; Embryos, Galaxies, and Sentient Beings: How the Universe Makes Life; Homeopathy: The Great Riddle; On the Integration of Nature: Post-9/11 Biopolitical Notes;* and *Migraine Auras: When the Visual World Fails.*

CALM HEALING CD

Methods for a New Era of Medicine

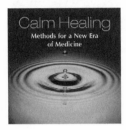

Practice of Deep Release—
The Practice of Self-Care: 26:18 minutes
Breathing Healing Energy—
Vase Breathing: 21:44 minutes
Using Inner Light—
Reversal of Suffering: 7:12 minutes

Text: Robert Bruce Newman
Voice: Charles Carreon

$19.95, ISBN 978-1-55643-635-2

Available from the Medigrace website at
www.medigrace.org:

ALZHEIMER'S CARE

Audiocassette (MG5)

Healing Within: 16 minutes
Inner Peace: 20 minutes

$17.95

NEAR DEATH CARE

Audiocassette (MG2)

Healing Through Hearing in Unconscious States: 26 minutes
Liberation Through Hearing After Death: 27 minutes

$17.95

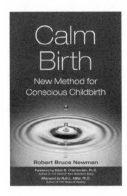

CALM BIRTH

New Method for Conscious Childbirth

Robert Bruce Newman
Foreword by David B. Chamberlain, Ph.D.

$15.95, TRADE PAPERBACK, ISBN 978-1-55643-612-3, 228 PP.

CALM BIRTH CD

Empowering Preparation for Childbirth

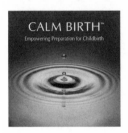

Practice of Opening: 22:15 minutes
Womb Breathing: 22:12 minutes
Giving and Receiving: 12:21 minutes

Text: Robert Bruce Newman
Voice: Dara Knerr
Music: Michael Mish

$19.95, ISBN 978-1-55643-588-1

CALM MOTHER CD

Empowering Postnatal Self-Care Methods

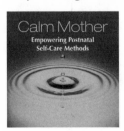

Calm Mother: 20 minutes
Sitting into Energy Body: 20 minutes
Breast-Breathing, Breath Feeding: 13 minutes
Practice of Healing: 14 minutes
Calm Parents: 11 minutes

Text: Robert Bruce Newman
Voice: Kari Marble
Music: Michael Mish

$19.95, ISBN 978-1-55643-636-9

For more information about the Calm Birth program, products, and services, please visit the Calm Birth website at www.CalmBirth.org.